D1411818

This book is dedicated to my father
GILBERT HENRY MEINZ
1922–1978

In his living he taught me the foundations of a
successful life. In his dying he not only solidified my
passion for promoting health but also brought me to a
higher level of understanding in my Christian faith.
I look forward to seeing my dad again.

This book is written for the glory of my heavenly
Father. He has given me my purpose in life and every
good thing I need. I pray that this book will help
others not only to maximize their health, but to also
realize the timeless wisdom of God's Word.

Acknowledgments

Many individuals contributed to the successful completion of *Eating By The Book*. Among those, I'd like to especially thank Dr. Charles Wickman, who gave me the personal and theological encouragement to pursue this project. Dr. Jeffrey Levin introduced me to the vast amount of research on the faith and health relationship. To my editor, Lila Empson, and my researcher, Ellen Sayed, my heartfelt thanks. Dr. Bryan Haddock, Dr. Garrett Kelley, Judy Doherty, Ann Volpe Daley, Ray Overton, III, Barbara Robidoux, and Nancy Brinn all helped to enhance the quality of this project as well. And finally I want to acknowledge Stan Martin, MA, who entered and reentered the manuscript into the computer untold times. Thank you for your input and all the hours. I will forever be amazed at your grasp of the rules of English grammar.

Go to
www.DavidMeinz.com
and sign up for your FREE
e-Health Newsletter

Plus, get your
FREE COPY of David's
*Fast Food Hall of
Fame & Shame*

Table of Contents

Part I: The Fattening of America

Part II: The Biggest Killer

Part III: Cancer: Prevention Is the Best Medicine

Part IV: The Secrets of the Pyramid

Part V: What The Bible Says About What You Eat

Table of Figures

About the Author

Nutritionist David Meinz claims it's not what you eat between Christmas and New Year's that matters but what you eat between New Year's and Christmas! He speaks internationally to businesses, associations, churches, and religious organizations and is a frequent guest on radio and television, including *Focus On The Family* and *The 700 Club*. Meinz's formal education includes a master's degree in human nutrition (MS) from the University of Missouri. He is also a registered dietitian (RD).

Meinz has been a full-time professional speaker since 1991 and has earned the Certified Speaking Professional (CSP) designation in the National Speaker's Association. He is also a fellow of the American Dietetic Association (FADA), an honor held by less than one percent of all dietitians. He is the only individual in the world to hold both designations. Meinz has taught nutrition at the university level, worked in human nutrition research and clinical dietetics, and was director of a hospital health promotion program.

As a Christian and a dietitian, he was pleased to discover that many of the current scientific recommendations on health and nutrition closely follow the Old Testament dietary laws. Just as a person's spiritual health can affect their physical health, David also believes that a person's physical health can positively impact their spiritual health as well.

He believes that physical health and *prevention* of illness have, for the most part, been overlooked by the Church. David believes it is better to stay well than to be healed. While spiritual health is, of course, of the highest importance, he points out that the Bible teaches that our earthly vessels have value and importance as well. He reminds his audiences that Jesus ministered to people's spiritual needs most often by also ministering to their physical needs.

The Bible teaches that our bodies are a temple of the Holy Spirit. David feels a strong calling to help people apply this truth to their daily lives.

Introduction

You Came with an Owner's Manual

Would you like to feel better, lose some weight, lower your cholesterol, and get fit?

Do you believe in the Bible? Do you believe that the wisdom found within it's pages still applies today?

If so, *Eating By The Book* may be what you're looking for.

According to scripture, God's plan for you is that you live your life *abundantly* (John 10:10). Most would agree that having good health is a big part of that abundance.

In *Eating By The Book* you will be challenged and encouraged. Challenged to consider the application of God's Word regarding your health today. Encouraged by the discovery of simple, practical steps you can take to maximize the health of your body that is so fearfully and wonderfully made. You'll learn how to lose weight and keep it off. You'll also learn how to prevent the two biggest killers of Americans today. And finally, you'll discover what the Bible specifically has to say about what your family eats for dinner tonight.

We don't need science to confirm God's Word, but isn't it nice when the secular world finally starts to catch up to the truths of the Bible? In just the last several years scientific research is beginning to make a case for the benefits of faith. Everything being equal, it appears your religious faith can have a profound effect on your health. In over 200 studies that have looked at the role of religion and health, the conclusions suggest a strong relationship.

> In over 200 studies that have looked at the role of religion and health, the conclusions suggest a strong relationship.

For example, a study at Dartmouth Medical School found that heart surgery patients who drew comfort and strength from their faith had a death rate three times lower than those who did not. Another study of 400 hospitalized heart patients discovered that intercessory prayer may actually work. (As believers we know it does, but to get the world to acknowledge that there might actually be something there is amazing.) In the 10-month study, half the patients had people praying for them, the other half did not. The half being prayed for, incidentally, *did not know* they were being prayed for. Those receiving prayer needed less medicine and had lower blood pressure, less congestive heart failure, and fewer heart attacks!

Isn't it interesting that God tells us in Matthew 18:19 "Again, I tell you that if two of you on earth agree about anything you ask for, it will be done for you by my Father in heaven."

A review of the scientific literature shows that the influence of religious faith can also result in

- **Reduced blood pressure**
- **Increased survival rates**
- **Less alcohol, cigarette, and drug use**
- **Less depression, anger, and anxiety**
- **A greater sense of happiness and well-being**
- **Greater marital satisfaction and stability**
- **Less stress and fewer psychological problems**
- **Better self-esteem**

Now, some might argue that those with religious beliefs are healthier because their religion prohibits or discourages their involvement in dangerous activities like smoking and using drugs. While that certainly may be part of the answer, your body doesn't care *why* you're not smoking—it simply appreciates the fact that you're not! Even so, studies that factored out these dangerous lifestyle habits *still* found a protective effect from faith.

In other words, researchers compared religious people who smoked with atheists who smoked and still found that the people of faith had better health! In spite of that faith, however, the health experience of many Christians often looks very similar to that of nonbelievers because their lifestyles are not that much different from the world's. The grocery cart of a Christian looks about the same as that of someone who has never opened a Bible. That's too bad, because God's Word has *a lot* to say about what you eat.

When Moses came down from Mount Sinai God gave His people these simple commandments for life (Exodus 20:3–17):

Jehovah's Top Ten List

1. You shall have no other gods before me.
2. You shall not make for yourself an idol in the form of anything in heaven above or on the earth beneath or in the waters below. You shall not bow down to them or worship them. . . .
3. You shall not misuse the name of the LORD your God, for the LORD will not hold anyone guiltless who misuses his name.
4. Remember the Sabbath day by keeping it holy. Six days you shall labor and do all your work, but the seventh day is a Sabbath to the LORD your God. . . .
5. Honor your father and your mother, so that you may live long in the land the LORD your God is giving you.
6. You shall not murder.
7. You shall not commit adultery.
8. You shall not steal.
9. You shall not give false testimony against your neighbor.
10. You shall not covet your neighbor's house. You shall not covet your neighbor's wife, or his manservant or maidservant, his ox or donkey, or anything that belongs to your neighbor.

Not a bad list. Do you know of a better set of rules to live by? Would even nonbelievers benefit from following them?

As Christians we are now, in fact, saved from the curse of the law. But it still shows us what God desires in our life. If we are indeed born-again Christians, then our desire should be to please the Lord. If the law shows us what pleases God, then surely our desire should be to do what pleases Him. But not out of obligation so much as out of joy and thankfulness!

Jesus said he came not to destroy the law but to fulfill it (Matthew 5:17). But that word "fulfill" has an unfortunate sense of completion or finality about it. A better interpretation of the original Greek word is to re-establish or re-affirm. When Christ came he confirmed the law as the standard of righteousness.

It is not legalism to desire to follow God's law. Legalism is trying to establish your righteousness with God outside of Jesus Christ.

The Ten Commandments are from the Old Covenant. Jesus Christ is the New Covenant. But those commandments are still as beneficial today as when they were first given 3,500 years ago. Imagine what a different world we'd have if people everywhere made their daily decisions based on these ten guidelines to life.

Would the United States have one of the highest murder rates of any industrialized nation in the world? Not if everyone practiced "You shall not murder," and "You shall not covet." If people didn't lie as a matter of course in everyday modern life, this world would be turned upside down! Time and time again, God continues to prove the timeless nature of His Word.

> Time and time again, God continues to prove the timeless nature of His Word.

What you eat or don't eat certainly has *nothing* to do with your eternal life. If you've accepted God's gift of Jesus Christ as your only means of salvation, then according to the Bible you *are* saved. *Period.* Hopefully the actions you take after receiving that salvation will reflect the new person you've become. But it's clear that modern-day Christians are no longer spiritually bound to the Old Testament dietary laws.

However, you may still get physical benefit from following those dietary laws! Our bodies, our digestive systems, and the enzymes that break down our food are basically the same today as they were when Abraham was alive. The human body has not changed that much in 3,500 years. Christ's resurrection changed the nature of our spiritual relationship with God, but it didn't change the nature of our physical bodies.

Someday we will have a new temple, but right now we have the old-fashioned kind, the kind that gets sick, the kind that dies. Our spiritual relationship with God no longer requires us to follow the dietary laws, but we may still want to because of the truth and wisdom of the Old Testament. When we as New Testament believers apply that truth and wisdom today, we can expect to benefit by doing so.

God's wisdom never ends. And just as an automobile owner's manual tells us how to work on a particular model, God's Word tells us how to work on the human model. There has never been a better guide for living life than the Bible. It shows us how to be a better spouse, parent, and businessperson. It tells us how to handle our money, our anger, our sorrow, and our joy. God's owner's manual also reveals how to experience the abundant health that God wants for His children.

PART

I

THE
FATTENING
OF
AMERICA

1

How I Lost 112 Pounds in Just One Week

Made you look! If you're still in the bookstore, this is probably the page you turned to first. Lose 112 pounds in one week? Sound impossible? *It is impossible!* You'd never fall for a claim like that, would you? Yet we fall for the equally ridiculous claims that manufacturers are making for Miracle Diet Pills, Electric Exercisers, and Amazing New Grapefruit Weight-Loss Plans. If you really want to lose weight see Chapter 4.

In the meantime, it's important that you realize that promoters can say or claim just about *anything* on radio, TV and in the newspaper, and it doesn't have to be true! Many consumers believe that claims for new weight-loss programs must be legitimate or "they couldn't put it on television." Surely that full-page ad in the newspaper for the Magic Fat-Melting

Pill must be true or else the newspaper wouldn't run the ad.

Wrong, wrong, wrong! No government agency screens these ads and claims before you hear about them. These advertisements don't have to get cleared by anyone. TV stations, radio stations, and newspapers are free to run just about anything as long as the client has the money to pay for it.

Because of our first amendment right to free speech, people can basically say whatever they want in this country. They can claim that *up* is *down* and *black* is *white*. They can outright lie. And, as long as they don't slander someone or commit libel, they can get by with it.

The Federal Trade Commission (FTC) does have the legal power to stop false advertisements. But they don't have the budget or the manpower to follow up on more than just a few of the hundreds of complaints they receive. *Let the buyer beware* is the motto. If a weight-loss product sounds too good to be true, it is.

> If a weight-loss product sounds too good to be true, it is.

Obesity is not unique to our country or to this modern age. In Judges 3:15–30 we read of Eglon, the king of Moab, who ended up with a sword plunged into his belly. He was so obese that "even the handle sank in after the blade . . . and the fat closed in over it." In 1 Samuel 4:18 we find that Eli was so (old and) fat that when he fell backward he broke his neck. Too bad they didn't have access to all the "wonderful" weight-loss products of today.

Eighty million Americans go on a diet every year. We spend between $30 billion and $50 billion(!) on weight-loss products and services annually. If a dieter goes on a traditional restrictive fad diet he or she has about a 95 percent chance of gaining all of the lost weight back, and even then some, within five years.

In this country the average person gains weight with age.

Now that doesn't mean it's okay to gain weight with time, it just means that it's the *average*, that most people do it.

The average weight gain for men in their 30s is four pounds. For women, it's nine pounds. But now, in addition to this average weight gain, Americans are putting on more weight above and beyond what we have seen in the past. Americans are not only getting fatter with age, as did their parents, but they're adding even more weight on top of that as well.

A 50-year-old weighs more today than a 50-year-old did 20 years ago. A 30-year-old weighs more now than a 30-year-old did 20 years ago. The number of Americans who were seriously overweight remained steady in the adult population for a number of years. In 1980, 25 percent of Americans were overweight. But that number has grown in the last few years to 65 percent. Over half of the adults in this country—about 100 million—are overweight!

The percentage of youngsters who weigh too much is growing too. About three times as many children and teenagers today are overweight compared to their counterparts 20 years ago. Enrollment in daily physical education classes in high school went from 42 percent in 1991 down to 28 percent in 2003.

> **O**ver half of the adults in this country—some 97 million— are overweight.

While not all overweight children become overweight adults, the tendency is there. Over half of our adult population is overweight today, even though most of them didn't start out that way as children. With the increase in excessive weight gain in childhood, the next generation may have an even greater epidemic of this problem. Will *all* Americans be overweight someday?

Americans are becoming more and more overweight for

the same two reasons they always have. First, they're eating too many calories—especially too many calories from fat and sugar. Second, Americans are physically inactive. In the old days people had to open the barn door by hand; there were no automatic garage door openers. They had to actually walk up stairs, not take an elevator. They had to hitch horses up, not just turn a key in the ignition. Those little things added up, and represented a much more active lifestyle than we have today. Our lives have become so high-tech and filled with labor-saving devices that we don't even have to get up off the couch to change the television channel. You may work hard at the office and be exhausted when you come home at the end of the day. But your work activities are probably not the kind that take fat off your body. Most Americans need to eat less fat and become more physically active in their lifestyle.

2

What's So Bad About Being Overweight?

Obesity's contribution to heart disease, high blood pressure, stroke, cancer, and other problems kills 300,000 people in this country every year. But you never hear anyone say, "He died from obesity." The death certificate usually ignores the influence of having too much body fat.

Heart Disease

Since heart disease is the number one health threat in this country, it's important to identify those factors that will increase the risk of suffering from this killer.

Adding fat to your body can, over time, dramatically contribute to your chances of having a heart attack. Excess weight will cause problems with your blood cholesterol numbers, increase your blood pressure, have a bad effect on your blood sugar levels, and contribute to a number of other problems as well.

Fat that accumulates around your waist appears to raise your risk of a heart attack far more than fat that accumulates on your hips. As you've probably observed, men tend to store more of their excess fat around their stomach. That's one more reason why obesity in men is more dangerous than in women.

High Blood Pressure

As you increase weight, you increase your risk of having high blood pressure. That's a fact. High blood pressure, also called *hypertension*, is the most common long-term disease in the United States. Some 50 million Americans suffer from it. High blood pressure alone contributes to 700,000 deaths every year from heart disease, stroke, and kidney disease.

A recent study found that the best way to lower blood pressure is to lose body fat. Surprisingly, the research found that blood pressure that is lower because of weight loss was not dependent upon whether or not patients were restricting their salt intake at the same time. It's also been observed that a person's salt-sensitivity—that is, the ability to handle salt without getting high blood pressure—can improve as weight is brought back closer to normal. In other words, if you are one of the salt-sensitive people and your blood pressure does go up when you eat more salt, that problem may go away as you get your body weight under control. It's estimated that up to 50 percent of all the adults in the United States who are currently on blood pressure medicine could get off of it completely if they were to lose only

> High blood pressure alone contributes to 700,000 deaths every year from heart disease, stroke, and kidney disease.

a little weight. It's important to realize that you don't *ever* have to get to your "ideal" body weight. Research shows you can experience a remarkable improvement in your health by taking off as little as 10 percent of your current body weight.

Diabetes

As your excess weight goes up, so does your risk for diabetes. And diabetes, in turn, contributes to your risk of heart disease. Once again, the *location* of your excess body fat seems to be important here too. Obesity in your midsection increases your risk for diabetes more than does excess body fat around your hips or on other parts of your body.

Cutting your calorie intake can dramatically improve your blood sugar control, even before weight loss has a chance to happen. Here's another example where lower-fat eating can help. You can decrease your calorie intake without having to decrease the *amount* of food you take in every day. How? By eating a lower-fat diet that is based on whole-grain complex carbohydrates like whole wheat breads, cereals, pastas, and related foods. As you'll soon see, your calorie intake will go down when you eat lower-fat foods closer to the way they were designed. If you reduce your calorie intake you have a good chance of better control of your blood sugar levels. However, be aware that *very* low-fat, *very* high-carbohydrate intake can be potentially dangerous for *some* people with diabetes. But we're not promoting those extremes. It's just that some people take things too far. The recommendations in *Eating By The Book* are good for diabetics too. A registered dietitian is your best source of specific dietary information if you have diabetes.

Arthritis

As your weight goes up, so does your risk for osteoarthritis. Excess body weight can put real stress on your knee joints, and that often is where osteoarthritis appears. A study found that obese women had almost four times the risk of osteoarthritis as normal weight women. For men, the risk was almost five times as much. People in the highest 20 percent of weight categories have seven to ten times the risk of having osteoarthritis as those in the lowest 20 percent.

Osteoporosis

Osteoporosis affects greater than 25 million people in this country over the age of 45—most of whom are women. Every year more than half a million women past the age of menopause have their first fracture of the vertebra of the spine. A million more fractures occur every year in people who already have osteoporosis.

Our theme throughout *Eating By The Book* is that *moderation* is the foundation upon which nutrition and good health are built. And a great example of that is in the effect that body weight has on osteoporosis—the brittle-bone disease. This is one of the very few, if not the only example, where excess body fat may actually have a more protective effect than having too little. What? Good news about being overweight? Don't get too excited.

For a long time we've observed that women who are overweight have fewer problems with osteoporosis. That's right. *Fewer problems.*

Any weight-bearing activity like walking or jogging causes the bones to become stronger. The stress of exercise sends a message to the bones to become stronger and more resilient in order to meet the challenge of the exercise. That's why we recommend some kind of weight-bearing exercise to all women.

It now appears that a woman who has been overweight for some time has unknowingly been doing weight-bearing exercise simply by walking around every day. Even though she may not be doing any formal exercise at all, her bones react by becoming stronger.

Being overweight also seems to protect women from

osteoporosis because excess body fat causes greater production of estrogen and other hormones that all help to maintain bone mass. Additionally, since many bone fractures occur as a result of falls, women with excess body fat frankly have more of a cushion to protect themselves when they do fall. A thinner woman experiencing the same type of fall might break a bone.

Ironically, thinner women who have watched their weight all their life by overly restricting calories may also have consumed a diet that was inadequate in nutrients like calcium. As a result, they often don't have the good bone density that would help to prevent osteoporosis.

So what should you do? Should you consider carrying around some extra body fat to prevent osteoporosis? No. The protection that you might get from carrying around extra body fat can't begin to compensate for the increased risk

Excess body fat may actually *help* protect a woman from osteoporosis.

you'll have from other health problems. You may cut your risk of osteoporosis, but you'll simultaneously *increase* your risk of heart disease, diabetes, and high blood pressure. Besides, body weight is only one factor that influences your risk of osteoporosis.

Maintaining good nutrition, exercising, and possibly taking the right medications, *is* the most effective approach to preventing and treating osteoporosis.

Endometrial and Breast Cancer

The same weight level that decreases your risk for osteoporosis *increases* the risk for endometrial cancer. That excess weight results in a two to three-and-a-half times greater risk.

Heavier women are not only more likely to get this cancer of the uterus, but they are more likely to die from it once they do have it.

Women who have too much fat on their bodies are also at greater risk for getting postmenopausal breast cancer—and for dying from it. And while it appears that fatter women seem to have a *decreased* risk of *pre*menopausal breast cancer, when they do get it, the time before the breast cancer recurs is shorter, and their chance of survival is less than that of normal weight women.

> The location of your fat seems to have an effect on your risk.

In obese women who haven't yet gone through menopause, therefore, breast cancer is deadlier than in more normal weight women of the same age.

And once again, *where* that fat is located seems to have an effect on your risk. Compared to fat on your hips and thighs, fat around the middle section of your body increases your risk of postmenopausal breast cancer. And if you have a family history of breast cancer, midsection body fat increases your risk of breast cancer even more.

Colon Cancer

Cancer of the colon is the second most fatal form of cancer in the United States; only lung cancer kills more. Up to half of all cases of colon cancer in this country seem to be due to an inherited family tendency. But for the other half, other factors are involved. These factors include lifestyles that are low in physical activity and diets that are high in fat, high in calories, and low in fruit and dietary fiber.

Some studies seem to imply that increased body weight increases risk for colon cancer; the vast majority of current research, however, does not support that theory. What we do know is that being overweight may be linked to insufficient physical activity and a high-fat, low-fiber eating pattern. Even though excess weight itself may not increase the risk for colon cancer, the presence of that excess weight may be a good indicator that other risk factors are involved.

Prostate Problems

In a recent Harvard study of over 28,000 men between the ages of 40 and 75, researchers discovered that men whose waist measurements were greater than 43 inches were more than twice as likely to have enlarged prostate glands as were men whose waists measured 35 inches or less. It's not your weight that's predictive of this, but where that weight is located. And, once again, it's that abdominal fat that increases the risk for an enlarged prostate.

How does this happen? There are several possibilities. Abdominal body fat actually increases estrogen production in men (yes, men do produce estrogen), and lowers testosterone levels. Too much estrogen is believed to irritate the prostate gland. Also, as we've said, higher than normal body weight can cause higher blood pressure. That higher blood pressure may also irritate the prostate. Researchers have not yet determined whether losing abdominal fat decreases the risk of prostate problems; it is clear, however, that men whose weight is closer to normal are more likely to avoid this problem.

Your Pocketbook

Not only does being overweight increase your risk for the biggest killers in this country, it also contributes to the cost. Every year we spend about $39 billion (that's $39,000 million) on coronary heart disease! The price tag for adult-onset diabetes is $19 billion; for high blood pressure, $12 billion; and for gall bladder disease, $10 billion. Couldn't we put those "sick-care" dollars to better use somewhere else?

Obesity

As if all these complications from being overweight weren't bad enough, it now turns out that being fat increases your risk of getting fatter still! The fat on your body is actually stored in tiny fat cells. The average-weight adult has some 30 billion of them. These cells expand or contract, depending on how much you weigh.

> **B**eing fat increases your risk of getting fatter still!

Scientists used to believe that your body had created all the fat cells you'd ever have by the time you reached adulthood. They thought that if you gained weight your fat cells got bigger and that if you lost weight they got smaller.

Researchers have now discovered that when you exceed about 60 percent of your ideal weight, your body actually starts creating more fat cells! This means that your body now has the capacity to become even fatter than ever before. It's as if you were to build a second story on your house. With one floor your home can hold just so much furniture. But if you build a second floor you can put a lot more in. You've still got just one house, but its capacity for storage has expanded tremendously. A very obese person may go from the average of 30 billion up to as many as 100 billion fat cells—all ready and willing to store even more fat. The fatter you get, the fatter you can get.

3

Just How Fat
Are You?

I don't own a bathroom scale, and you shouldn't own one either. That sounds like heresy in a society that seems to worship the bathroom scale. Most weight-loss programs say you're successful when the scale goes down. I disagree.

The Liar Scale

Do you ever get up in the morning and stand on the bathroom scale to see what kind of day you're going to have? If the scale goes up, you're going to have a miserable day. If the scale goes down a pound or two, you're happy.

The doctor's office height-and-weight table has been used for decades as "the standard" to determine your health status in relation to weight. It didn't attain that status because it was so accurate; it's just been used unquestionably because we didn't have anything else more reliable.

The scale in your bathroom or in your doctor's office

measures your *weight*—period. The scale will tell you how many pounds you're contributing to the weight of the Earth. That's all. Your weight doesn't necessarily measure the status of your health. We now know that *what your weight is made up of*—fat, muscle, or water—is far more important than your total weight.

If your scale says you've lost 10 pounds, that really tells you very little. Did you lose 10 pounds of fat? If so, good for you. If, however, you went on a traditional crash diet by cutting back on food and ignored exercise, those 10 pounds weren't just fat. Most likely, your weight loss was a combination of some fat, a couple of pounds of muscle, and the rest was water.

The bathroom scale is a liar.

The scale can't report anything but *weight* loss. It can't tell you how much fat you lost. It can't tell you how much water you lost. It can't tell you how much muscle you lost. It just tells you the total from all three. On a crash diet, because your kidneys are working overtime, you may find yourself going to the bathroom frequently. You only need to lose two cups of water to lose a pound of weight on the bathroom scale. That's why it seems so easy to lose weight so quickly. That's why you can lose a couple of pounds over the weekend. You didn't lose body fat; you lost water. You trusted the scale when it seemed to say, "Congratulations, you lost weight." In fact, you lost water weight. The scale is a liar.

When you get off that crash diet and start eating normally again, you'll put that water weight back on equally as fast. When the scale goes back up you'll think you're getting fat again. No you're not. You're getting rehydrated!

The next time someone says they lost four pounds over the weekend, ask them if they want a glass of water. Since you can look at them and see they didn't get skinny, they must just be *dry*! If someone loses 10 pounds of something and asks your help in finding it, you'll want to know specifically what you're looking for. If a scale tells you you've lost 10 pounds, it doesn't tell you anything except 10 pounds, period. You need more information than that.

The Height-and-Weight Table

A muscular football player standing six feet tall and weighing 225 pounds would be overweight according to the height-and-weight table. A football player's body is heavier than that of the average person of the same height—but it's not *fatter*. Why? Because muscle weighs a lot more than the same amount of fat. Since so much of this football player's weight is muscle, his body ends up being heavier than the average person his height. And yet using the height-and-weight table, the traditional advice would be for him *to lose weight!* From where? He barely has any fat on him in the first place. The only way to get to his so-called desirable weight would be to lose muscle tissue, which would accomplish nothing except hurt his health.

The height-and-weight table can also *under*estimate body fatness. It could indicate, for instance, that your weight is perfectly appropriate for a person your height, and yet you could still be fat. How's that possible? As we age we tend to

> The average inactive person loses about five pounds of muscle per decade.

lose muscle and gain fat. The average inactive person loses about five pounds of muscle per decade. Even if you've stayed the same weight since high school, you may have lost muscle and replaced it with an equal amount of weight from fat. That's why former high school football players can brag that they weigh the same as they did twenty-five years ago—but can't begin to get into the old uniform. Fat takes up more space than an equal weight of muscle. And since muscle has been replaced with fat, the measurements of these former athletes expand. Once again, the bathroom scale is a relatively useless piece of equipment.

Another problem with the height-and-weight table is that it represents information collected on people who have insurance. Since that doesn't necessarily reflect everyone, the predictions of health and longevity implied in the tables may not necessarily be dependable. Many people who are within the ideal weight range end up with poor health and suffer early death. Conversely, many people whose weight falls outside their ideal range enjoy good health and live a long time. The height-and-weight table also makes it appear that being thin is dangerous to your health. But the table doesn't take into account the fact that many thin people who die were simultaneously smoking cigarettes or otherwise ill. In general, thinness doesn't threaten your health. Rather, diseases and disorders that lead to thinness threaten your health. If these problems were factored out, desirable weights for height would be even more conservative than they are now.

The height-and-weight table has many shortcomings. Fortunately, some new approaches can more legitimately link your weight to your long-term health prospects.

BMI

Body Mass Index (BMI) is a mathematical ratio of your height to your weight. It's becoming a popular way of defining your weight because health professionals now only have to use a single number to learn a lot about your current health status. The well-respected Framingham study has indicated that if everyone met the ideal range of these guidelines, there would be 25 percent less coronary heart disease and 35 percent fewer strokes in this country.

Research is showing that a body weight that corresponds to a BMI of 23 in men and a BMI of 21 in women is ideal. Someone with a BMI between 25 and 29 is considered officially overweight, and his risk of health problems is increased. A man within this range who also has a waist measurement of greater than 40 inches is at an even higher risk for problems. A woman with a BMI between 25 and 29 with a waist measurement of more than 35 inches is also at a higher risk.

A BMI at or above 30 officially qualifies as obesity. Once again, a man whose waist measures more than 40 inches or a woman with a waist measurement of more than 35 inches significantly increases his or her potential for even more health problems.

> Even if you have a lot of weight to lose, going down just one or two BMI units can dramatically reduce your risk of health problems.

Experts are now suggesting that if your BMI is above 25, you should concentrate on losing one or two BMI units and then maintaining that level for about six months to a year. After allowing your body to get used to this new weight, try to lose another one or two units and repeat the maintenance phase.

This approach may increase your chances of keeping weight off for the long term. Even if you have a lot of weight to lose, going down just one or two BMI units can dramatically reduce your risk of health problems. Blood cholesterol numbers can improve and blood pressure can go down. And if you suffer from arthritis, decreasing your weight only two BMI units can significantly decrease your symptoms as well. Besides, it's much easier to successfully take off *one* or *two*

BMI units than it is 50 pounds.

Build on slow, positive success. Keep in mind that you didn't gain all that weight overnight. You don't have to take it off that quickly either.

Even though the BMI is an improved measure for the vast majority in determining where you are and how you're improving, it has its shortcomings. It's not applicable for children, pregnant or breastfeeding women, serious bodybuilders or frail elderly. You can also have a desirable BMI reading and still need to lose weight if your waist measurement is larger than it should be.

What I don't like about the BMI is that you have to use the scale to measure your progress. You will still always want to know how many *pounds* you've lost. You'll still want to use that lying bathroom scale as your measure of success.

Body Fat Percentage

What you *really* want to know is how much fat you have on your body. There are now ways to indirectly measure your actual body fat as a percentage of your total weight. To do this you'll need access to the right tools.

Many health clubs and universities have skin-fold calipers, bioelectrical impedance analysis (BIA) devices, or underwater weighing equipment. In trained hands, all three of these can give you a good idea of your body fat percentage. I'd stay away from the relatively new infrared equipment, however. Its accuracy is questionable.

Underwater, or hydrostatic, weighing equipment can give a very good idea of how much fat you have and how much fat you're losing. Hydrostatic weighing is based on the principle that water and oil don't mix—and your body fat is simply another form of oil.

You're put into a big tank of water to see how easily you float. If you have a hard time staying under the water, you probably have a higher percentage of body fat. But if you sink

Figure 3.1

WHAT'S YOUR BMI?

Weight	Height															
(lbs)	5'0"	5'1"	5'2"	5'3"	5'4"	5'5"	5'6"	5'7"	5'8"	5'9"	5'10"	5'11"	6'0"	6'1"	6'2"	6'3"
120	24	23	22	21	21	20	19	19	18	18	17	17	16	16	15	15
125	24	24	23	22	22	21	20	20	19	19	18	17	17	17	16	16
130	25	25	24	23	22	22	21	20	20	19	19	18	18	17	17	16
135	26	26	25	24	23	23	22	21	21	20	19	19	18	18	17	17
140	27	27	26	25	24	23	23	22	21	21	20	20	19	19	18	18
145	28	27	27	26	25	24	23	23	22	21	21	20	20	19	19	18
150	29	28	28	27	26	25	24	24	23	22	22	21	20	20	19	19
155	30	29	28	28	27	26	25	24	24	23	22	22	21	21	20	19
160	31	30	29	28	28	27	26	25	24	24	23	22	22	21	21	20
165	32	31	30	29	28	28	27	26	25	24	24	23	22	22	21	21
170	33	32	31	30	29	28	28	27	26	25	24	24	23	22	22	21
175	34	33	32	31	30	29	28	27	27	26	25	24	24	23	23	22
180	35	34	33	32	31	30	29	28	27	27	26	25	24	24	23	23
185	36	35	34	33	32	31	30	29	28	27	27	26	25	24	24	23
190	37	36	35	34	33	32	31	30	29	28	27	27	26	25	24	24
195	38	37	36	35	34	33	32	31	30	29	28	27	27	26	25	24
200	39	38	37	36	34	33	32	31	30	30	29	28	27	26	26	25
205	40	39	38	36	35	34	33	32	31	30	29	29	28	27	26	26
210	41	40	39	37	36	35	34	33	32	31	30	29	29	28	27	26
215	42	41	39	38	37	36	35	34	33	32	31	30	29	28	28	27
220	43	42	40	39	38	37	36	35	34	33	32	31	30	29	28	28
225	44	43	41	40	39	38	36	35	34	33	32	31	31	30	29	28
230	45	44	42	41	40	38	37	36	35	34	33	32	31	30	30	29
235	46	45	43	42	40	39	38	37	36	35	34	33	32	31	30	29
240	47	45	44	43	41	40	39	38	37	36	35	34	33	32	31	30
245	48	46	45	44	42	41	40	38	37	36	35	34	33	32	32	31
250	49	47	46	44	43	42	40	39	38	37	36	35	34	33	32	31
255	50	48	47	45	44	43	41	40	39	38	37	36	35	34	33	32
260	51	49	48	46	45	43	42	41	40	39	37	36	35	34	33	33
265	52	50	49	47	46	44	43	42	40	39	38	37	36	35	34	33
270	53	51	50	48	46	45	44	42	41	40	39	38	37	36	35	34
275	54	52	50	49	47	46	45	43	42	41	40	38	37	36	35	34
280	55	53	51	50	48	47	45	44	43	41	40	39	38	37	36	35
285	56	54	52	51	49	48	46	45	43	42	41	40	39	38	37	36
290	57	55	53	52	50	48	47	46	44	43	42	41	39	38	37	36
295	58	56	54	52	51	49	48	46	45	44	42	41	40	39	38	37
300	59	57	55	53	52	50	49	47	46	44	43	42	41	40	39	38

Healthy Range: 19–24   Overweight: 25–29   Obese: 30+

easily, you may have a good amount of muscle and a lower, healthier amount of body fat. While you're in the water you'll be weighed and a technician will determine how much fat and muscle you have on your body.

The problem with this most accurate method is that it's rather cumbersome. Not only do you have to blow all the air out of your lungs, you then have to stay completely submerged under water for what seems like an eternity. It's actually only about 15 seconds, but a lot of people find they can't do it.

Skin-fold calipers and bioelectrical impedance devices are a lot less traumatic than underwater weighing and will still give you a good idea of how much body fat you have. In the meantime you can use Figure 3.2 on page 29.

The Tape Measure

Since researchers have discovered that fat around and above your waist is far more dangerous than fat on your hips and thighs, your waist-to-hip ratio (WHR) is a very good way to determine your weight and fat status. All you need is an 89¢ tape measure.

WAIST/HIP RATIO
$$\frac{\text{Waist Measurement}}{\text{Hip Measurement}} = 0.8 \text{ or less}$$

To calculate WHR, simply divide your waist measurement by your hip measurement. Your waist should be measured at the halfway point between the top of your hipbone on the side and the bottom of your rib. Your hip measurement is taken at its widest point. A ratio of 0.8 or less is best.

For example, if you measure 37 inches in the waist and 35 inches in the hips, divide 37 by 35. Your WHR would be 1.1, well above the desired goal of 0.8.

Figure 3.2

GAUGE YOUR BODY FAT

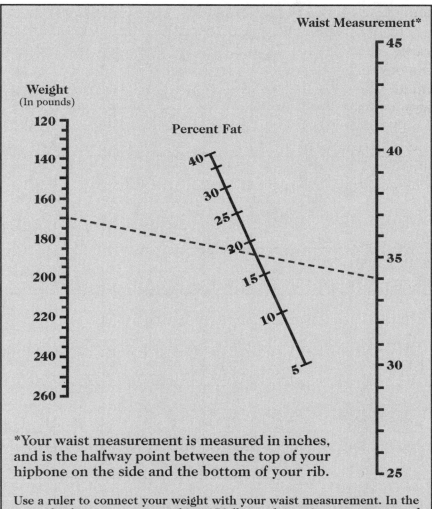

Waist Measurement*

Weight
(In pounds)

Percent Fat

*Your waist measurement is measured in inches, and is the halfway point between the top of your hipbone on the side and the bottom of your rib.

Use a ruler to connect your weight with your waist measurement. In the example above a person weighing 170 lbs. with a waist measurement of 34 inches would have approximately 18 percent body fat. The reading on the middle line is a quick *estimate* of your body fat percentage. And what goal should you be aiming for? A healthy level for women is 18–21 percent of their total body weight as fat. For men, 16–19 percent. At these levels you will look great and be contributing to good overall health.

Reprinted by permission from J. Wilmore, 1986, Sensible Fitness. 2nd ed. (Champaign, IL: Human Kinetics), page 30.

Figure 3.3

MEASUREMENTS PROGRESSION RECORD

	DATE	NECK	WAIST	ABDOMEN	HIPS	MID-THIGH	TOTAL INCHES LOST IN THIS 3 MONTH PERIOD
BEGINNING MEASUREMENTS							
3 MONTHS							
6 MONTHS							
9 MONTHS							
12 MONTHS							
15 MONTHS							
18 MONTHS							
21 MONTHS							
24 MONTHS							
GRAND TOTAL OF INCHES LOST							

Remember, the tape measure is your best choice to document decreasing body fat as you progress in your program.

This is worth repeating. Carrying more fat around the waist increases your risk of heart disease, high blood pressure, breast and endometrial cancer, high cholesterol, and diabetes.

In the Harvard study referred to earlier involving 28,000 healthy men, it was found that those with waist measurements of 40 to 68 inches were five to 17 times more likely to develop diabetes in the next five years than those who had waist measurements of 27 to 34 inches.

If you measure your success in weight loss with a tape measure, you'll not only document your improved waist-to-hip ratio, but you can also monitor your overall inches lost as well. When the tape measure goes down, the fat is going down too.

Use the Measurements Progression Record, Figure 3.3, to monitor your progress over the next two years. Two years? Yes, two years. Body fat that you take off slowly is much more likely to stay off. Our goal is to get you off of diets *once and for all*.

4

How to Lose Weight and Keep it Off

When it comes to losing weight, there's a lot of information available. There's a lot of *mis*information available, too. What you should be interested in is what will work over the *long term*. If you want *quick* weight loss there are plenty of choices. But you've probably been down that road. You don't want quick—you want *permanent*.

In the past you *may* have been able to cut back on calories, which worked all right for a while. But you found, eventually, that even when you followed the diet perfectly and didn't cheat, the weight loss slowed down and even stopped.

What's worse, every time you went on a new diet the weight not only came back but you gained a little extra as well. You ended up weighing more than you had before you started the diet! Frustrating.

The answer to successful permanent fat loss is not in a magic pill. You won't find it in some miracle product on a late-night infomercial, either. The right way to lose inches and fat is incredibly easy to understand—and for most people incredibly hard to accomplish. To take off your excess fat and keep it off involves three straightforward steps.

We've known about these steps for some time now; no overnight revelations here. But you don't hear about them very often because they don't involve much glamour or glitz. No Hollywood movie star is promoting this approach.

In fact, some people find the fundamental foundation that the three steps are based upon downright unappealing. What is that foundation? *Self-responsibility.* Many people aren't ready to take on that role. They'd rather continue in the lifestyle that got them fat in the first place and just wait for the latest artificial sweetener or fat substitute to come along. Surely the latest discovery about the fat gene in mice is the answer they've been looking for.

> A recent study at Purdue University revealed that churchgoers are actually *more* likely to be overweight than those who don't attend.

In the meantime they get fatter and fatter waiting for the next magic pill. People are dying at epidemic rates from diseases directly related to obesity. Lives and ministries are often cut short because Christians stumble in this one particularly personal area.

If, on the other hand, you're one of the few who are ready to acknowledge that you can do "everything through him who gives me strength" (Philippians 4:13), and if you are willing to do what it takes to regain the good health with which God graciously blesses most of us in the beginning of our lives, then read on.

How to Lose Weight and Keep it Off
Step Number One: Eat Less Fat and Sugar

For some time the official recommendation for good health has been to aim for no more than 30 percent of your calories coming from fat per day. Of all the calories you eat, about a third of them should come from fat; the rest should come from carbohydrates and protein.

There never was anything magical or scientific about this goal. It simply seemed like a good target since many Americans were eating about 40 percent or more—far too many— of their daily calories from fat.

A number of health authorities today suggest a goal of even lower than 30 percent. I agree.

Let's talk percentages. I don't think you should spend much time concerning yourself with the fat percentages listed on a product's nutrition label.

First of all, percentages can be confusing. Many people still think the recommended daily fat intake is 30 *grams*. After all, that's the number they've been hearing for years. But grams and fat percentage are not the same thing. Thirty grams of fat is *not* the same as 30 percent fat!

Second, fat percentage can also be misleading. A product can have a lot of fat and still have a relatively low fat percentage if it also contains a lot of sugar.

Finally, it's all so unnecessary. Keeping a rough running total of how many grams of fat you eat for breakfast,

> **T**hirty *grams* of fat is not the same as 30 *percent* fat!

lunch, and dinner accomplishes the same goal in a much more straightforward manner.

Over the last two decades Americans have decreased the percentage of their calories coming from fat from about 37 percent to the current 34 percent. That sounds good. But in fact, most Americans are actually eating the same or even slightly *more* fat than 20 years ago. And that's in spite of all the emphasis on low-fat foods! How can our percentage intake have gone down when our consumption has gone up? Simple mathematics.

We are now eating more *total* calories than before, much of which is due to an increased sugar consumption. Our average total daily calorie intake has gone up from 1,800 calories in the 1970s to 2,100 calories today. As total calories go up, the percent contribution that fat makes to the total obviously decreases.

But your body doesn't care about percentages! Your body is affected by the *total* amount of fat you're eating every day. The average American will eat about 82 grams of fat today. That's way too high for most of us. My recommendation is simply to consume 50 grams of fat a day or less. True, for some people that's on the conservative side. With an average intake of about 2,100 calories in a day, 50 grams of fat comes out to be 22 percent of calories from fat.

> The average American will eat about 82 grams of fat today.

But is that a problem? Can you go too low in your fat intake? You really don't have to be concerned about getting *too little* fat. No one is dying today from a fat *deficiency*. People *are* dying from eating too much fat. Besides, some evidence is showing that the amount of fat needed to help prevent certain cancers may be less than the often recommended 30 percent level. In general, the less fat you take in, the easier it is to also control your calorie intake and your weight.

With a little effort, and the suggestions in *Eating By The Book*, you can live comfortably on 50 grams of fat a day. Going much below that, however, may be too difficult to fit into your routine, and the scientific evidence doesn't really show any health benefits from going below this conservative intake. Nevertheless, if you're an average American and the only change you make in your diet is to start eating around 50 grams of fat a day, chances are very good that you'll lose weight.

> E at 50 grams or less of fat per day.

We eat too much sugar too. Way too much. A lot of it comes from soft drinks. In 2000, the average American drank 53 gallons of bubbled sugar-water! I hardly drink any at all, so that means somebody out there is not only drinking theirs' but my 53 gallons too. By the way, only about one-fifth of soda consumed is the sugar-free version. If you want to make an impact on calories, cut your soda consumption down. You may be surprised what an impact that one step can make on your waistline.

But when it comes to losing inches and body fat, the most effective thing you can do is to limit your dietary fat intake. Here's why.

Why You Should Eat Less Fat
Strike #1
Nothing Has as Many Calories as Fat

By design, food is either protein, carbohydrate, or fat. That's it. Any food you've ever eaten or ever will eat has to fit into one of those three categories.

In the United States we normally think of getting protein from lean meats.

Carbohydrates, also called starches, include potatoes, pastas, rice, breads, and cereals. Fruits and vegetables are also carbohydrates.

Fats come from animal fat on meats, cooking oils, butter, margarine, mayonnaise, sour cream, and deep-fried foods, to name just a few. Compared to protein and carbohydrate, fat has over *twice the calories* per serving.

Ounce for ounce, gram for gram, fats have over twice as many calories as anything else you'll ever put on your plate. Per ounce, even sugar—a carbohydrate—has less than half the calories of fat. A teaspoon of sugar has 16 calories. But a teaspoon of butter or traditional margarine has 35 calories!

> Ounce for ounce, gram for gram, fats have over twice as many calories as anything else you'll ever put on your plate.

Yet many people believe sweets like candy are just as "fattening" as greasy foods like onion rings. They have been told since they were little, "Carbohydrates are fattening. Watch out for all those potatoes and breads and starches — you'll get fat!" In fact, carbohydrates have the same number of calories per unit volume as protein. And you never hear anyone saying that protein is fattening! The people who told you that carbohydrates and starches were fattening didn't mean to mislead you—they were just passing on misinformation that someone else told them.

Consider this: When you eat a plate of spaghetti, you know you've had something to eat! You feel full. Why? Because carbohydrates/starches *take up room* on your plate and in your stomach. You get satisfied with the meal. Carbohydrates fill you up but they don't fill you out. When you start eating more carbohydrates—breads, potatoes, cereals, pastas—you'll be pleasantly surprised how much food you get to eat and *not* gain weight.

If you want to cut calories, don't cut out the potatoes, don't cut out the pastas, and don't cut out the proteins. Instead, eat less of the fats, the butters, the margarines, the sour creams, and the deep-fried foods. Since there's over twice the number of calories in a serving of a fat food than in an equal serving size of a carbohydrate or a protein food, when you decrease fat you automatically bring down the calorie level.

A good weight-loss program doesn't necessarily have to include calorie counting. Please realize, however, that the *total* number of calories you take in is still important. Don't let anyone tell you otherwise. But when you count fat grams, you control both fat and calories at the same time. When you decrease fat grams, you can't help but bring the calories down. If you just count calories, however, you can potentially end up with a low-calorie, high-fat diet.

If you take a small baked potato, a carbohydrate/starch, at 100 calories and add one level tablespoon of fat, like margarine, what happens? You *double* the calories. That margarine takes the calories from 100 to 200. And let's be honest—for a lot of people one level tablespoon isn't enough for a whole baked potato; they use two or three tablespoons, and some people have even been known to add some sour cream—more fat.

> **W**hen you count fat grams you control both fat and calories at the same time.

Do you see how easy it is to take a small baked potato at 100 calories and turn it into 400 calories? And yet what gets the blame for being fattening? The *potato*. When people eat a steak dinner, one of the first things they'll push aside when trying to lose weight is the potato. "Oh, I'm cutting down on starches; pass the butter, please."

The fact of the matter is, while it's still on your plate—even before you eat it—*nothing* has as many calories as foods with fat.

You also need to realize that there is *no* controversy about whether carbohydrates are good for you or not. That issue has been settled. Carbohydrates are to be the foundation of what you eat every day. The food pyramid (page 180) is based upon this concept. In fact, the foods God originally gave us were carbohydrates, namely fruits and vegetables (Genesis 1:29). It was only after the flood that God allowed the higher protein meats and animal foods. If you go to any nutrition department at any legitimate university in this country, you'll get the same answer. Carbohydrates are good for you. Especially whole-grain, less processed carbohydrates. Period. End of discussion.

> The foods God originally gave us were carbohydrates.

So why do we *continue* to hear how fattening and bad carbohydrates are? Why do these low-carbohydrate (also called high-protein) diets make it to the best-seller lists? Because diet books continue to be among the most popular of all books year in and year out. And since most people don't want to buy a book that promotes self-responsibility, the authors of diet books have to come up with gimmicks.

In simplistic terms, God has designed your body to get energy from two sources: carbohydrates and fats. Some diet books claim that if you don't eat carbohydrates your body will be forced to just burn fat. That seems logical, but it's not true. Without the presence of carbohydrates in your diet, your body will only *partially* burn fat. Instead of using up your fat, your body produces ketones, a substance from the partly burned fat. Unfortunately, these ketones can lead to problems with your kidneys, blood pressure, and cholesterol levels. Additionally, they can be especially dangerous during pregnancy and can lead to brain damage and mental retardation in an infant. Nevertheless, these diet books continue to be very popular. Why? Because people *do* lose weight on a low-carbohydrate diet!

One side effect of the presence of these ketones is a decrease in hunger. You simply become less interested in food and your appetite goes down. You eat fewer calories, and the scale can go down too.

Additionally, when your body first detects a lack of carbohydrates in your diet, it starts using its own stored carbohydrates—called glycogen—found in your muscles and liver. Connected to that glycogen is water. When you burn the glycogen you end up going to the bathroom a lot to get rid of it. As you know, water is heavy and you can lose a lot of weight very quickly when starting a low-carbohydrate diet. That weight will come back on again, however, as soon as you start eating normally again.

Furthermore, your body does not like ketones and will send them out in your urine. Once again you're losing water, and the scale goes down some more. Many people on low-carbohydrate diets find themselves constantly thirsty and simultaneously going to the bathroom all night long.

So low-carbohydrate diets start out by making you dehydrated, not thin. You combine that with the fact

> Low-carbohydrate diets end up making you dehydrated, not thin.

that they are also low in calories (they don't tell you that), and people do end up losing weight on these fad diets. *But it doesn't stay off!* Remember, you can say or write anything in this country and it does not have to be true! Why do these books keep coming out? Because there's big money to be made. Nothing wrong, of course, with making money. But when it comes with a potentially high price tag to your health, there is something wrong with that.

The best advice I can give you is to stop falling for these quick fixes. The Bible tells us to "be as shrewd as snakes and as innocent as doves" (Matthew 10:16). If some new legitimate "diet breakthrough" is ever discovered, it will put the diet industry out of business, not contribute to it. People will get on it, lose the weight, and then be done with it. But don't hold your breath. In the meantime you have to ask yourself, if low-carbohydrate diets work, how come they didn't work years ago when they first came out? Why do we continue to have new versions of these fad diets every year? What happened to all of those people who claimed success in those earlier diet books? I'll tell you what happened to them—they're the ones buying the new diet books today. You can absolutely count on the fact that next year there will be another whole crop of diet books, and then some more the next year, and the next, and the next. Stop wasting your valuable time and your hard-earned money.

> **If low-carbohydrate diets work, how come they didn't work years ago when they first came out?**

What's presented in *Eating By The Book* is not very earth-shattering. You won't find any miracle breakthroughs. But what you'll learn here *works*. Study after study has found that people who successfully keep weight off for years share two characteristics—they eat fewer calories (often by eating less fat) and, as you'll see, they put exercise into their lifestyle. What you're learning in *Eating By The Book* is commonsense, scientifically-based information. The fact that it fits in with God's Word helps too.

Why You Should Eat Less Fat
Strike #2
There's No Limit to the Fat You Can Store

As long as you keep eating fat your body will be happy to accommodate you. Eventually, you'll accommodate yourself right into a bigger wardrobe! The body basically has an unlimited amount of room to store fat. All you have to do is think about those 500–600–700–pound people you see on television and you know it's true.

By God's wonderful design He created the human body with the ability to store extra food when it was readily available. Then, if times got lean or if a famine hit, an individual could continue to live off their fat even though food was scarce.

What an incredible invention this human body is! It's like having a car with an unlimited gas tank. You can buy gasoline when it's 99¢ a gallon and just drive around for months on that and not worry if the price goes up to $3.50 per gallon or if there's a fuel shortage. You don't care—you've got plenty.

Even though fat storage is basically unlimited, your carbohydrate and protein storage *is* quite regulated. Carbohydrate is stored in your muscle cells and liver in the form of glycogen. Your body can only store a grand total of about 1,700 calories in the form of this carbohydrate. When you accumulate more than that you simply have no more room.

In the past we believed that extra calories from *any-where*—fat, carbohydrate, or protein—would eventually turn into fat on your body. While it's true that laboratory rats and hibernating animals can turn extra carbohydrate into fat, new research is suggesting that we humans, for all practical purposes, cannot. So what happens to those calories?

It appears that as you eat more carbohydrates your body becomes more efficient in burning them up! The more bread, cereal, and pasta you eat, the quicker the body burns them.

> In the past we believed that extra calories from *anywhere*— fat, carbohydrate, or protein— would eventually turn into fat on your body.

If you turn the temperature in your oven from 300° up to 450° whatever's inside will get burned faster. When you eat more carbohydrates you are, in effect, turning up your oven and burning carbohydrate calories faster.

I know this may be a new concept to you, it's a new concept to me too. The prestigious *American Journal of Clinical*

> **I**n the form that God created them, it's very hard to gain weight on carbohydrates.

Nutrition recently dedicated an entire issue to new findings in carbohydrate metabolism. It revealed that if the carbohydrates you eat are in the form that God created—*whole* grain, as opposed to simple carbohydrates like sugar—and you're eating an average-calorie, well-rounded intake of nutritious foods, *it's very hard to gain weight on carbohydrates!*

The story is basically the same for protein intake too. Americans eat an average of about 80 grams of protein per day. With four calories in each gram, that comes to 320 calories from protein. Unlike fat and carbohydrate, protein doesn't really have *any* storage form at all. If you eat a lot of protein your muscles don't get bigger! Only if you're doing serious resistive exercise like weight lifting, will your body add protein to your muscles.

After you reach your protein needs for the day your body once again—just as it did with carbohydrates—becomes more efficient in burning up the extra protein you eat.

How quickly you burn up excess dietary carbohydrate and protein is determined by how much of each you take in. The more you eat, the quicker they're burned. The rate that fat is burned, however, does not have such a control mechanism in humans. In general, the more fat you eat, the more fat you store.

Of course, all of this is not license to go wild with calorie consumption!

As we've said, the total number of calories you consume is important. Some research shows that if you are in a constant state of being overfed (look up to see what God said about gluttony in Proverbs 23:2), you will actually *decrease* your body's ability to use fat as an energy source—during exercise, for example.

Now don't be intimidated by all of this biochemistry. *Remember that you accumulate fat on your body by overeating fatty foods—not by overeating complex, whole-grain carbohydrates or protein.*

Why You Should Eat Less Fat
Strike #3
Fat Directly Contributes to the
Two Biggest Killers

As we've said, the two big killers in this country are heart disease and cancer. Remember, too, that food is only made up of three different substances: protein, carbohydrate, and fat.

The amount of protein that you eat—like lean turkey without the skin, for example—is not related to your risk of heart disease. The amount of protein you eat is also not related to the risk of cancer.

The amount of carbohydrate that you eat is not related to your risk of getting heart disease or cancer either. Even the carbohydrate called sugar is not the problem. While sugar can cause tooth decay, and diabetics certainly have to be careful of excessive intake of sweets, sugar still doesn't entirely deserve the bad reputation it has.

But, the amount of fat you eat—especially animal fat, called saturated fat—*is* related to your

> Only fat is related to both heart disease and cancer.

risk of both heart disease and cancer.

So, of the three categories of food—protein, carbohydrate, and fat—and the two main sources of death in this country—heart disease and cancer—only fat is related to both the number one and number two killers. And *that* is strike number three in our case against fat.

We don't need to stop eating fat altogether, but we do need to cut down on how much we eat and how often we eat it. To summarize the case against dietary fat: Strike #1—Ounce for ounce, gram for gram, and pound for pound, fat has over twice the calories as either carbohydrates or protein. Strike #2—You body has an unlimited ability to store fat. Strike #3—Only fat directly contributes to today's two biggest killers in America.

How to Lose Weight and Keep it Off
Step Number Two:
Put Physical Activity into Your Lifestyle

Most Americans love sports. Actually they love *watching* sports. In fact, 60 percent of all Americans don't get the recommended amount of regular physical activity they need. In addition to that, 25 percent get no activity at all. Only 15 percent consistently get at least three good aerobic exercise sessions per week.

Do you have to run marathons to be healthy? No! In fact, you don't have to run at all. You can begin by walking. I'm not talking about taking a social stroll; I'm talking about engaging in a serious activity. But a brisk walk that requires you to swing your arms and really move down the road may be all you'll ever need. Brisk walking, stationary bicycle, aerobics class, square dancing, roller skating; whatever you want to do is fine, but choose something that's *fun* for you. Exercise doesn't have to be a chore to be good, and more is not always better.

Research is now showing that lighter exercise results in many of the same health benefits as all-out fitness training. In fact, marathon runners often are more likely to come down with a cold or flu during their intense training periods than those who exercise at a more moderate level.

Interestingly, scientists are getting mixed results on the benefits of swimming. Some research shows that swimming doesn't seem to be as effective as exercises on land for body fat loss. While some ideas exist, researchers aren't entirely sure why that is.

Make no mistake. Swimming is great for your cardiovascular fitness to improve your lungs and your heart. If you're overweight and really out of shape, swimming is a great place to start. Your chances for injury are minimal, and most people with excess body fat find exercising in the water an enjoyable experience. Nevertheless, for long-term body-fat loss, some studies suggest that other types of exercise may be more efficient. To be on the safe side, for serious body fat loss choose something other than swimming.

What does exercise really accomplish? Yes, activity does burn calories. But that's not the only reason you should exercise. Actually, exercise is rather inefficient in burning those

> To lose that one pound of body fat you'll have to run the equivalent of 35 miles!

calories—you have to run about a mile to burn 100 calories.

Let's say your weight is perfect except you're just one extra pound heavier than your ideal weight. To lose that one pound of body fat you'll have to run 35 miles!

That's rather depressing isn't it? Here's the bottom line. While the calories you burn during *aerobic* exercise can add up over time, one of the main purposes of activity during a weight-loss program is to protect your muscle tissue. When you decrease the number of calories you're consuming, your body tries to make up the difference from several different sources. First is from body fat, which is what we want. But your body can also burn muscle for calories. You never, never, never want to lose muscle tissue! Why? Because that's where you burn a lot of your calories every day, especially during exercise. Physical activity protects muscle tissue while the body burns fat.

> You never, never, never want to lose muscle tissue!

On the other hand, if you're on a weight-loss program and do not exercise you'll burn muscle too. If you start out as a six-cylinder engine, you may eventually become a four-cylinder. Your "machine" will get smaller. As a result, when you go to bed at night you won't be burning as many calories just lying there as you did before you began your diet. That's not good.

Instead of *losing* muscle you need to *increase* your engine size; take your six-cylinder and make it into an eight-cylinder. People who never do any exercise can, with time, actually become little two-cylinder engines with such lowered metabolisms that they can hardly eat anything without gaining weight. Don't decrease your engine size, increase it. The main thing you want to do with exercise is to protect that muscle tissue and make it more efficient. And if you can actually *build* the muscle tissue, then you can increase your metabolism even more.

Exercise helps do that, especially *resistive* exercise where you're working with Nautilus or Universal machines or with some type of weights. When you gain muscle tissue you increase your metabolic rate. You burn more calories every day—just by living! Those extra calories can really add up. Some researchers have found a greater decrease in body fat and increase in muscle tissue when resistive training is the exercise of choice. My recommendation is that you do both resistive and aerobic.

Aerobic exercise also increases the number of enzymes that allow the fat to leave their cells. As we've said, the fat on your body is made up of billions of individual fat cells, each one of which contains enzymes that allow fat to go in and different enzymes that allow stored fat to come out. When you integrate regular exercise into your lifestyle you'll increase the number of the fat-releasing enzymes. As a result, the fat can then more effectively get back into the blood and down to the muscle cells to be burned up for energy. Additionally, aerobic exercise will also cause your muscles to more effectively use that fat once they receive it.

This means that three months into an exercise program you'll be *more* able to use body fat as your energy source for the exercise than you could when you first started. Energy to exercise comes from two places—blood sugar and blood fat. As exercise becomes part of your lifestyle and you continue to exercise week after week, your body will develop a greater ability to get that energy from fat. More of the calories you burn in exercise will now be coming from fat and less from blood sugar. Now you'll not only lose pounds, but you'll more effectively lose *inches*, and *that* is what weight loss is all about—not what the scale says, but what the mirror says.

> Three months into an exercise program you'll be *more* able to use body fat as your energy source for the exercise than you could when you first started.

Start out with some kind of aerobic activity like walking briskly (on a treadmill or otherwise) or riding a stationary bicycle. Three months later, add a resistive exercise of some kind.

If you do both types of exercise in the same day, do your aerobics first so you get the blood flowing and the muscles warmed up. When you finish your aerobics, cool down for a few minutes before doing your weight lifting routine. And women, this is not just for men. Exercise benefits you just as much as it does men in terms of long-term weight control. And you don't have to worry about bulking up. You won't end up looking like a female version of Arnold Schwarzenegger. That's probably just fine with you anyway.

What specifically should you do? Start with a 5 to 10 pound weight for your upper body and maybe 30 to 40 pounds of weight for your lower body. Use some kind of light weights or a safe piece of equipment at a gym or your local recreation center. You can even get resistive exercise machines in home models too.

Lift the weight that you can do comfortably for 8 to 12 repetitions. When 12 repetitions become too easy, either increase the weight slightly or increase the number of repetitions. Work on major muscle groups like your arms, chest, back, abdominals, upper legs, calves, and shoulders.

Can you exercise and just forget about nutrition? Without

Your Creator did not design you to sit for extended periods of time in an easy-chair!

making serious changes in your diet it appears that exercise alone will not result in a significant change in your body weight or your body fat content. Make no mistake. Exercise is an *absolute necessity* for long-term weight control. That can't be overemphasized. Your Creator did not design you to sit for extended periods of time in an easy-chair!

But research is also showing that without combining activity with decreased fat and calories, you may get very fit—that is, your heart and lungs may become more efficient—but you won't get thin. Exercise that's followed by a high-fat meal seems to be a waste of time. Which is more important, exercise or nutrition? Both are most important!

How to Lose Weight and Keep it Off
Step Number Three:
Throw Your Scale Away

Crash diets limit your food choices. You may be "allowed" lettuce, cottage cheese, and all the celery you want. You may be told to avoid carbohydrates since they're "fattening." Exercise? Don't worry about it. You can lose weight without it.

And can you lose weight on a crash diet? Yes! You can lose weight simply because crash diets severely limit your caloric intake.

And does the weight stay off? Absolutely not!

Since crash diets don't require you to change the lifestyle habits that got you fat in the first place, as soon as you finish the Miracle Grapefruit Weight-Loss Plan the pounds come back.

But let's say, instead, you do everything right. You *do* eat less fat. You *do* put physical activity in your lifestyle. You're perfect! Nevertheless, if you do *everything* right but fail to throw out your bathroom scale, you may *still* miss your success.

The bathroom scale only tells you weight loss, not what that weight loss is made up of! When you correctly remove fat from your body you'll lose inches, your waist will get smaller, and your dress or pants size *will* go down. But the scale may not go down as much as you'd expect.

Let's say as a result of successfully following the first two steps for body fat loss that you have lost 10 pounds of fat and your inches have gone down too. But since you've also integrated physical activity—especially resistive exercise—into your lifestyle, you're building muscle at the same time. As

Figure 4.1

FAT TAKES UP MORE ROOM THAN MUSCLE

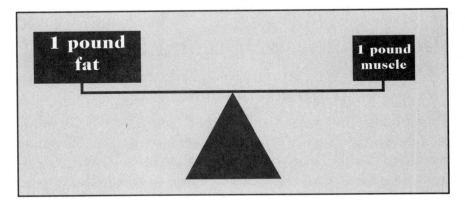

we've said, we know muscle weighs more than fat per unit volume since a pound of muscle takes up less room than a pound of fat.

If you lose 10 pounds of fat but, because of physical activity, gain seven pounds of muscle, the liar scale will say you've only lost *three little pounds!* The scale can't tell you what the weight loss is made up of. You're wearing smaller clothes, you're looking great in the mirror, and all your friends want to know your secret—but the scale says you're a failure. And if you believe the scale you *will* be a failure.

You must free yourself from the addiction to the bathroom scale. If after all the work you've done you think you've only lost three pounds, you'll quit. I'd quit too. But the fact is that you're an incredible success story. You look better and you feel better. You've accomplished what most people just dream about. And you'll throw it all away if you believe the bathroom scale.

I have to reluctantly admit here that the best long-term study of people who have lost significant weight and keep it off has shown that they, in fact, do monitor themselves. Most often with the scale. But they're not obsessive about it and many just weigh on a weekly basis. It certainly isn't the reason for their success. They use the scale to help themselves from sliding back into their old habits.

I maintain you could do the same thing with a tape measure. Fat takes up room and if your dress or pants start getting tight again that tells you all you really need to know. I'm going to stick with my position that the bathroom scale does more harm than good. My advice is that you don't depend on it to tell you what's really going on during your effort to lose body fat.

> You must free yourself from the addiction to the bathroom scale.

Figure 4.2

THE WRONG WAY TO LOSE BODY FAT

THE RIGHT WAY TO LOSE BODY FAT

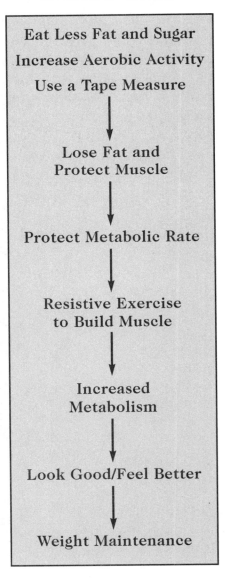

Fad Diet

Don't Exercise

Use the Scale

↓

Lose Muscle

↓

Decreased Metabolism

↓

Look Bad/"Drawn Out"

↓

Eat Even Fewer Calories to Maintain Weight Loss From Lower Metabolic Rate

↓

Possible Malnutrition/ Poorer Health

↓

Eventual Weight Gain

↓

Repeat The Cycle

Eat Less Fat and Sugar

Increase Aerobic Activity

Use a Tape Measure

↓

Lose Fat and Protect Muscle

↓

Protect Metabolic Rate

↓

Resistive Exercise to Build Muscle

↓

Increased Metabolism

↓

Look Good/Feel Better

↓

Weight Maintenance

5

The FIT Formula

As you begin a program to lose fat and keep it off, you'll want to find some type of exercise you can integrate into your lifestyle. Remember, it's always a good idea to check with your physician to make sure you don't have anything in your medical history that would prevent you from participating at the level we discuss.

Of course, you want to be sure to warm up before exercising. It's important to get the blood circulating in your muscles to prepare for the intensity of your exercise session. If you jog, start with a walk. If you walk, start with a less intense stroll. On my stationary bicycle I pedal at a nice, low level for about five minutes before I start the actual exercise session.

When you're finished, be sure to ease back down by doing a less intense version of your exercise for a five-minute or so cool down.

An easy way to remember how often, how hard, and how long you should exercise is by thinking of the acronym FIT: Frequency (how often you should exercise), Intensity (how hard you should work out), and Time (how long your sessions should be). The following guidelines represent the most efficient fat burning formula.

Frequency

Frequency is the first key factor in fitness. The official recommendation in many circles today is to get 30 minutes of moderate physical activity *every day* for good health. That's fine, but I don't think most Americans will do it. You definitely need to do *something*, but exercising every day *for the rest of your life* is a little too overwhelming. For serious, long-term body fat loss your goal should be to exercise at least four times a week. For general cardiovascular health, your goal should be to exercise three times a week.

If you want to do more, that's fine. But I don't think it's practical for most people. If your goal is to exercise six days a week and you only exercise four, you may feel like a failure. But if your goal is to exercise four days a week and you're able to do that nearly every week, you'll be building on success. Realize that you don't have to be perfect in any of this. But for fat loss you should average at least four sessions a week, week in and week out, from now on. That's why it's so important to find some activity that you can realistically do.

If you have the time to exercise every day that's great. Most of us, however, have enough to do in our busy lifestyle without trying to fit daily exercise into an already overloaded schedule.

Intensity

Intensity is the second key factor in fitness. How hard do you need to exercise? For some time now, people have been given a specific calculation to figure their target heart rate (THR). The goal was to work up to a specific number of heartbeats per minute, which, in turn, reflected the correct intensity of exercise.

We now know, however, that target heart rate doesn't accurately reflect intensity level for as much as 40 percent of our population. That's a lot. While THR is still okay for the other 60 percent, there's no way to know if you are part of that majority. You may be exercising at an intensity that puts you right in your THR range and still be doing so at a level that's not particularly productive for you.

As an alternative, the best advice for most of us now is a simple three-step process: Exercise at a level where your heart is pumping faster, break into a sweat, and do it intensely enough that you're breathing more heavily but not so much that you get out of breath.

You should still be able to talk while you're exercising, but you shouldn't have so much wind that you can actually sing (maybe you can't sing anyway!). Or if you're exercising with a friend, your breathing should be faster and deeper than normal, but you should still be able to carry on a conversation—but not sing a duet!

If your exercise is so easy that you have enough breath left to sing, you need to push a little harder—walk a little quicker,

INTENSITY
- Faster heart rate
- Break a sweat *
- Never out of breath

*Incidentally, although most of us will, some people just don't perspire much—even at high intensities of exercise. That's probably okay, but talk to your physician to be sure.

swing your arms a little higher, or peddle a little faster. Within a couple of sessions, you'll get a feel for what intensity is a good one for *you* specifically.

On the other hand, you never want to exercise so hard that you get out of breath. Safety is an issue, of course, but there's something even more. An adequate amount of oxygen is required to burn body fat. When a fire has its oxygen supply shut off, it goes out. It's very similar in the cells of your body. If you don't have enough oxygen, the cells' ability to metabolize fat is severely limited.

When you exercise too intensely and get out of breath,

you run out of oxygen. When this happens, your respiratory and circulatory systems can't send the oxygen where the body needs it. As your oxygen supply decreases—when you *really* start huffing and puffing—you dramatically cut down on your ability to use fat as an energy source. So slow down!

The unchanging, fundamental concept of weight loss is that the more calories you burn the more weight you'll lose. Obviously, the harder you exercise, the more calories you'll burn. The harder you exercise, however, the shorter your exercise session will have to be. It's true that you'll burn more calories per minute, but you won't be able to keep on going as long.

> As your oxygen supply decreases you decrease your ability to use fat as an energy source.

You'll burn more calories at a moderate intensity for 30 minutes than you will from 10 minutes at a higher intensity that you can't maintain. Besides, the goal of exercise is not to push you to the point of exhaustion, but rather to become a part of your normal routine—something that you enjoy and find energizing.

Within the *good range* of intensity, however, there's some controversy regarding just how hard you should exercise. Some will say that lower intensity *aerobic* exercise utilizes fat on your body better than higher intensity *aerobic* exercise does, and there's some evidence to back that up.

But even though the *percentage* of fat used may be greater at a lower aerobic intensity, the *total* amount of calories burned during the exercise session is not as great as the total amount of calories burned at a higher level of intensity.

Of course, if you exercise for a longer time, a lower intensity exercise can certainly still have a good effect. Lower intensity, of course, is recommended for people just starting out on their activity program.

As your fitness level improves you should be able to exercise a little harder and still not get out of breath. When you do, you're becoming more efficient at burning fat too.

Time

Time is the third key factor in fitness. A good eventual goal for the length of your exercise session is around 30 minutes.

Interestingly, research is now suggesting that even shorter exercise sessions, just 10 minutes or so, done more frequently on the same day, can still give good cardiovascular and weight loss benefit. But will Americans, most of whom don't get the minimum three sessions *a week*, commit to three or four mini-sessions *per day* instead? I don't think they will. As we've said, most people have too many things going on. If you can, good for you. You're certainly better off doing three 10-minute sessions a day than not doing anything at all because you can't find a 30-minute slot. My advice is to do your exercise all at one time. Get it over with and get on with the rest of your day.

But what if you haven't exercised since Gerald Ford was president? What if the last exercise tape you listened to was an eight-track? What if the mere *thought* of 30 minutes of exercise causes you to become anaerobic?

If you're a little bit out of shape, you may only be able to do five minutes of exercise before you start to get out of breath. That's okay. You don't have to get in tip-top shape in the next week or so. As a matter of fact, you *don't ever* have to get in tip-top shape.

> You *don't ever* have to get into tip-top shape.

Research indicates that those who benefit the most from an exercise program are people who go from no activity to just a moderate level. What you need, however, is consistency. Increase your time slowly. If you can do five minutes now, a month from now you'll be doing 10 minutes quite easily. You might even be doing more than that.

Don't do too much at once. Give yourself some time to get to your goal. Consider where you're coming from! How long did it take you to get out of shape? Ten years? Twenty-five years? The fact is it will take you a *much* shorter amount of time to get back into shape. That's a pretty good deal if you think about it. You may have been getting out of shape for the last several decades. It may take you a year or two to get back into shape. That's not a bad deal.

As you increase duration, you can increase intensity as well. And frequency? Start with one or two days a week and work up to three or four.

Even though the emphasis here is on how to *decrease* body fat, the bottom line is that prevention is still the best medicine. Most people gain weight from their 20s to their late 60s. It may be average, but it's not good. One of the best things you can do to prevent *future* weight gain, regardless of where you are now, is to integrate good, effective physical activity into your lifestyle. As important as exercise is in the *treatment* of weight control for long-term success, it appears that it has an even

THE FIT FORMULA

FREQUENCY:
3–4 times per week

INTENSITY:
• Faster Heart Rate
• Sweat
• Stay Aerobic

TIME:
30 minutes

greater effect on keeping fat off of your body in the first place. Whether you're already at your goal or not, the very best way of making sure that exercise will be effective for you is by following the FIT Formula.

6

Here's Why You *Don't* Exercise

Like it or not, you *must* get some regular physical activity into your lifestyle. God designed you to *move.* That's why He put your legs so close to the ground! Researchers have found that a sedentary lifestyle is just as risky to your health as smoking a pack of cigarettes every day!

Some people say they're going to walk, and that's fine when the weather is nice. But what happens when it turns cold or rains or gets dark too early? All legitimate reasons, but no excuse. Excuses don't do anything to take and keep fat off of your body. You know you *should* exercise, you know it's good for you and you feel better when you do it—so why haven't you put fitness into your lifestyle? It's my experience that most people don't integrate activity into their routine for two reasons; inconvenience and boredom.

'Exercise Is Inconvenient'

As a speaker, I travel a lot. When I finally get to my hotel room or return home late, the last thing I feel like doing is rushing to a gym and waiting in line for a piece of equipment. If you're typical, your lifestyle doesn't allow you a lot of free time, either.

If you've ever said to yourself, "I *would* exercise if I could only find the time," here's how to solve that problem. First, do away with the inconvenience. I bought a piece of good quality home exercise equipment. Now, even if it's 8:30 at night, I can fit fitness in at *my* convenience.

That one step has made all the difference in finally integrating activity into my lifestyle again. No more rushing to the gym, changing clothes, and trying to fit into someone else's schedule.

I also discovered that I can never *find* time; I have to *schedule* the time. Every Sunday, I look at my calendar for the upcoming week and schedule three time slots for exercise. If someone calls and wants to meet with me at one of those times, I simply explain that I have an appointment. You don't have to tell people what you're doing at that time any more than you need to explain the rest of your schedule.

> You will never *find* the time to exercise.

All good intentions aside, if you don't plan for activity, other very legitimate needs will crowd it out. Saturday is going to come around anyway. By scheduling your exercise, you chalk up another week where you integrated positive, productive fitness into your life rather than once again being "too busy."

'Exercise Is Boring'

In this sensory-overloaded society of ours, sweating and grunting for a half hour doesn't appeal to too many people. I'm in the business of promoting good health. Yet even as much as I believe in the concept, I still didn't look forward to the drudgery of getting on my exercise bike. Talk about dull! Even reminding myself of how good this was for me didn't do it. The trick is to get your mind *off* of the monotony of exercise.

Here's what I did. I positioned my exercise bike right in front of the television, and that worked well for a while. But the commercials quickly put my mind back on the boredom. Instead, I now go to Blockbuster and rent a movie, but not just *any* movie. It needs to be one with *lots of action*—explosions and plenty of car chases. Schwarzenegger always helps too.

I start exercising, turn on the movie *Speed*, for instance, and my exercise session is finished before I know it! If my mind is on something else, the time flies. And here's an important point. When my exercise

> **Y**ou need to make fitness fun!

session is over, I shut the movie off and don't watch it again *until I get back on the bike!* As a result, I now have a built-in incentive to exercise again—because I want to see how the movie turns out!

Most movies are about 100 to 120 minutes long, and I get about three exercise sessions from each one. You might prefer to listen to a tape on your Walkman or watch a football game on television. The point is that you're looking for something that will make the time go by in an *enjoyable* way. Depending on where your attention is, your exercise session will either seem like an eternity or go by in a snap. *You need to make fitness fun!*

Find something that will fit into your lifestyle 12 months a year, something that you can realistically *stay with*. That's what it takes—*consistency*. It's not what you're able to do right after New Year's resolution time, but what you're still doing in May and July and next October.

This system works for me and it will work for you too. If you've been having trouble getting motivated to exercise, address the two reasons most people don't and you'll dramatically increase your chances for integrating successful fitness into your lifestyle.

Figure 6.1

BENEFITS OF EXERCISE

1. Reduced risk of developing heart disease, diabetes, colon cancer, and high blood pressure

2. Reduced blood pressure in those who already have developed high blood pressure

3. Increased utilization of fat as the energy source during exercise

4. Improved appetite control in those who are overweight

5. Increased muscle mass

6. Emotional lift

7. Normalized blood sugar

8. Increased HDL (good) cholesterol, decreased LDL (bad) cholesterol

9. Increased bone density

10. Decreased arthritis pain

11. Improved balance and muscular control in older adults

12. Increased long-term weight control

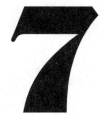

Methuselah Must Have Been Really Skinny

Most people in North America get fatter as they get older. Recently, some health professionals have suggested that the weight gain people experience with age should be considered normal. The traditional height-and-weight tables were actually changed a while back to allow more weight gain for people in their 40s, 50s, and 60s. When the seats in Yankee Stadium had to be replaced recently, they were actually made three inches wider than the old ones!

So, is getting fatter just a part of getting older? As a matter of fact, no. Many people who live outside of the Westernized countries maintain their weight as they get older. In some countries, people actually lose weight with age.

The well-respected Framingham study found that people who were 11 to 20 percent *under* the average weight for their height lived the longest. The National Institutes of Health agrees that the weights that are below average—as long as those weights are not associated with illness—are the ones associated with the greatest longevity.

> It may be possible to extend your life by as much as eight to sixteen years simply by paying more attention to the size of your waistline!

Scientists have known for years that mice and rats in middle age live 10 to 20 percent longer when they are fed all their required nutrients but at a lower calorie level. Studies using monkeys—a closer research model to humans than mice—also show the same thing. If this trend also turns out to be true in people, it may be possible to extend your life by as much as 8 to 16 years simply by paying more attention to the size of your waistline!

On the other hand, a study recently published in the *Journal of The American Medical Association* found that people who are overweight (BMI 25-29.9) but not officially obese (BMI 30 or more) actually have a *lower* risk of death than those of normal weight.

What's going on? Consider several issues. First of all, the differences in death rates between the normal and the overweight were not huge. So it doesn't make sense to put on a couple of pounds to just get into the overweight category. Secondly, the researchers included people in the study who had serious diseases such as cancer and heart disease; problems than can cause weight loss before death. By comparison, this can make bigger people who are not dying from a disease look healthier. And finally, and most importantly, the study only looked at death rates, not quality of life. We know for a fact that the more fat you have on your body the higher your risk of diabetes, gallbladder disease, high blood pressure, and lots of other problems that can effect your quality of life. So even if it turns out to be true that being a little overweight won't shorten your life, it may still negatively effect the quality of that life. The bottom line is that it's not OK to be overweight.

The Bible addressed this very issue long ago. Proverbs 23:20–21 says, "Do not join those who drink too much wine or gorge themselves on meat, for drunkards and gluttons become poor, and drowsiness clothes them in rags." Remember, Proverbs 23:2 says, "Put a knife to your throat if you're given to gluttony." Now there's the ultimate weight loss plan!

Have you ever seen an obese 100-year-old? Probably not. There's truth in God's Word.

We would never tolerate drunkenness in our church, but we often laugh about how much some people stuff themselves with food at church potlucks. Yet God puts drunkenness and gluttony on the same level. Ezekiel 16:49 says, "Now this was the sin of your sister Sodom: She and her daughters were arrogant, *overfed* and unconcerned. . . ."

Scripture says that only God knows how long each of us will live. King David said that longevity during his time was 70 years (threescore and ten). Our average life expectancy in this country has already surpassed that.

> The Bible says God *knows* the length of each person's life, not that he *determines* it.

If God knows how long we'll live, what difference does it make what we do? What difference does it make what we eat, or even if we exercise? Careful. The Bible says God *knows* the length of each person's life, not that He *determines* it.

My dad died from heart disease at the age of 56. Was that God's will? Was it God's will that my sister and I lost our dad?

Was it God's will that our mom lost her husband? God certainly knew when my dad would go to be with Him, but I think it was my dad himself who determined his length of life by the health decisions he had made during that life.

Consider this. If God indeed is the one in charge of the number of years you have, why don't you just jump off a building or step in front of a truck? If it's not "your time," you won't die. Right? And yet Scripture says we are not to put the Lord to the test (Matthew 4:7). Most people would never jump in front of a truck, but isn't that what we're doing when we carry an extra 40 pounds of fat on our body? Or smoke cigarettes? Or live an inactive lifestyle?

The number of years that God designed for the human body is *greater* than most people currently experience. Do you believe that God has a specific calling for your life? What if you retired at age 65 and still had another 30 vibrant years of good health to look forward to? Would that help you fulfill that calling?

Let's put things into perspective. For many people, just getting to your ideal weight—or, more appropriately, to your ideal BMI range—is a lifetime task in itself. To even consider going lower than that seems overwhelming.

The good news is that for most overweight people, taking as little as just 10 percent off your *current* weight will result in incredible improvements in your health. You'll decrease your risk for heart disease, diabetes, stroke, and cancer. You'll have more energy, you'll sleep better, and you'll improve your immunity. Don't underestimate the benefits of even the smallest long-term fat loss. Even Methuselah had to start somewhere.

> The number of years that God designed for the human body is *greater* than most people currently experience.

8

The Bottom Line

If you have a constant headache because you keep hitting yourself in the head with a hammer, an aspirin will help, but it doesn't deal with the cause. Until you get rid of the hammer, the aspirin is only a short-term answer.

Are you overweight because you simply don't understand the very basics of nutrition and fitness? Do you still think calorie counting is the answer? Although it's true that calories *do* count, today we realize there's a lot more to successful long-term weight control. If you need to learn the simple facts, *Eating By The Book* can help you. But for some people access to the facts is not enough. Getting rid of their "hammer" requires more effort.

Do you overeat because of emotional or spiritual issues? Do you eat when you're happy? Sad? Depressed? Angry? Lonely? Do you eat for emotional comfort? Food was never meant for that purpose.

God designed food for sustenance to keep the body alive and healthy. He also designed food for enjoyment. But God has not provided you with food to take the place of personal and spiritual relationships.

Do you overeat to avoid dealing with difficult issues? Do you believe that if you're not physically attractive you'll be safe from the advances of the opposite sex?

Were you raised in a home where food was given as a reflection of love? Was it implied that if you didn't take seconds you didn't really love the cook? Obviously there's nothing wrong with love, but food should have very little to do with it.

Emotional and spiritual reasons for obesity aren't related to nutrition or to a lack of exercise. They are related to what's going on inside your mind and spirit, which in turn manifests itself on your body. Under these circumstances, any weight you might lose will eventually be regained if the real cause is not addressed. A trained Christian counselor or pastor is the best first step you can take.

To successfully lose body fat you must be willing to change your lifestyle and change it *for the rest of your life*.

Yes, you need to eat less fat and sugar.

Yes, you need to find an exercise you *will* do about four days a week and do it for the rest of your life.

And yes, if it applies to you, you must be willing to deal with and correct any spiritual issues that may have put fat on you in the first place.

These are easy words to say, yet hard for the average person to carry out. But the average person doesn't have a clue as to the right way to get the job done—now *you* do! Remember, you can do *everything* through him who gives you strength! (Philippians 4:13)

> There's more to living than food—life is what you do *between* meals.

With both the knowledge and the power to get the job done, you now have the formula for long-term success.

ACTION STEPS
FOR WEIGHT CONTROL

1. **Stop falling for quick and easy "magic" weight loss plans.**
    Quit wasting your time and money. Get serious. Do it right
    once and for all and be done with it. You don't need to be
    on diets the rest of your life.

2. **Eat less fat and sugar. Eat 50 grams or less of fat per
    day.**

3. **Put physical activity into your lifestyle.** *Schedule* three or
    four fitness sessions a week and do something that is con-
    venient and FUN!!!

4. **Buy a tape measure and record the inches you lose.** Keep
    in mind that fat takes up room, but muscle weighs more.
    Successful fat loss will result in slower weight loss, but
    you'll look good in the mirror!

5. **Throw your bathroom scale AWAY!!!** Don't simply hide it
    in a closet. Don't simply stay off of it. Throw it away. If
    you don't, the scale will lie to you at your very moment of
    success.

6. **Decide if you're eating to live or if you're living to eat.**
    If you're using food as a replacement for something that's
    missing in your life, ask the Lord to help you put food
    in its proper place. Lots of help is available; take advan-
    tage of it. Talk with your pastor or a qualified Christian
    counselor.

Additional Resources
for Weight Control Information

Note: Please realize that much of what you find on the Internet today is *not* accurate
or trustworthy. This is especially true in the area of health. The Websites listed
in *Eating By The Book* have been reviewed and found to be dependable.

American Dietetic Association

Consumer Nutrition Hotline. Recorded messages and referrals to registered dietitians in your area. The largest group of certified nutrition professionals in the world. Reliable information from the nutrition experts.

 1-800-366-1655
 www.eatright.org

United States Government, National Agricultural Center, Food and Nutrition Center

Information on weight control and general nutrition.

 FNIC/NAL
 Room 105
 10301 Baltimore AVE
 Beltsville, MD 20705
 301-504-5719
 www.nal.usda.gov/fnic
 (select *fnic resource list*, and then *weight control.*)

National Institutes of Health

Scientifically-based information on weight control and nutrition.

 www.niddk.nih.gov

Under "Health Information" click on "Nutrition" or "Weight Loss." Also
visit the "Weight Control Information Network."

PART
II

THE
BIGGEST
KILLER

9

Fat's Where
It's At!

Fifty-eight thousand Americans died in the Vietnam War. That's the same number who die from cardiovascular disease in this country every three weeks! Yes, *every* three weeks.

In the next 21 days the number of people who will die from cardiovascular disease will equal the number who died in the entire nine years of the Vietnam war.

Then, three weeks after that, another 58,000 will die. And then another 58,000, and another 58,000, all year long, year in and year out.

And most of them are Christians.

> **P**reventing cardiovascular disease should be your number-one health goal.

The Korean War claimed 34,000 American lives. And yet that's the same number of lives that are claimed by cancer in this country every three weeks! Once again, 34,000 American lives cut short every twenty-one days. And then another 34,000 will die, and then another 34,000, every three weeks, all year long, year in and year out.

And most of them are Christians.

The United States still considers itself a religious nation. Eighty-two percent of the population identify themselves as Christians. Thirty-nine percent are born-again Christians. Heart disease and cancer kill more followers of Jesus every day than all the Roman gladiators ever did!

For every ten Americans, seven are dying from one of just two diseases. About 42 percent die from cardiovascular problems and about 25 percent from cancer.

> Heart disease and cancer kill more followers of Jesus every day than all the Roman gladiators ever did.

When my dad died on December 8, 1978, his death didn't make the front page of the newspapers. It didn't make it on the nightly news. And yet that one event tore my family apart, never to be the same again.

Multiply that story by a million and you can begin to see the devastating effect cardiovascular disease has on the United States *every year!* It's the number one killer. Nothing else comes close. Preventing atherosclerosis (what we used to call *hardening of the arteries*) should be your number one health goal. And the number one dietary contributor to the number one killer is fat in your food—especially animal fat.

If you're a typical American, odds are good that *heart disease* or *cancer* will appear on your death certificate as the cause of death. Statistically, the odds are that one of those is going to get you. But the *good news* is that you don't *have* to be a statistic!

The Bible says, "man is destined to die" (Hebrews 9:27), but you don't have to die early, nor do you have to get sick before you die. Wouldn't it be nice to live so long that your body simply wears out? We know that the human body can live around 100 years, but the average person still doesn't live anywhere near that long. Most people don't give their bodies a chance to wear out because their health habits allow some disease process to kill them prematurely. Make it your goal not only to extend your life to its full potential, but also to make your years healthy and productive ones as well.

Why die of heart disease if you don't have to? Resolve now to make changes in your lifestyle to prevent or treat this biggest killer of Christians.

10

Why Your Cholesterol Number Is Not Enough

You probably already know that the best way to bring down your blood cholesterol numbers is by eating less cholesterol and animal fat (also called saturated fat). You probably also know that the official goal for your cholesterol reading is 200 or less. But did you know that the average man who has a heart attack has a blood cholesterol level of only 223? Yes, only 223! The average woman who has a heart attack has a cholesterol reading of only 247. If you, like many people, think that 200 is the goal, you may also think that a reading of, say, 225 or 250 "isn't that far off." It's certainly not as bad as a reading of 300 or so.

The reality, however, is that more people have heart attacks with cholesterol readings *below 200* than those with cholesterols over 300! A reading "just a little above 200" is no reason to celebrate!

> **M**ore people have heart attacks with cholesterol readings *below* 200 than those with cholesterols over 300!

The current official recommendation of 200 milligrams per deciliter (mg/dl) or less for cholesterol is a little out of date. You're not *really* protected from heart disease until your reading is 150 or lower.

But the news isn't all bad. You may still be able to avoid heart disease even with a higher cholesterol number—if you have more information. Getting cholesterol tested with a finger prick at a shopping mall is not enough. Instead, ask your doctor to do a *total lipid profile* test. In addition to your total cholesterol level, this will also give you your HDL (the good cholesterol), the LDL (the bad cholesterol), and your triglycerides. The combination of that information will tell you far more than just getting your cholesterol number alone.

Your HDL (high-density lipoprotein) is good because it's the part of your cholesterol that's going through your arteries toward the liver and out of your body. The LDL (low-density lipoprotein) is bad because it's the part that deposits fat and cholesterol against your artery walls as it goes through. (Incidentally, the cholesterol in food is neither the good nor the bad kind. Cholesterol becomes good or bad only once it gets into your body. There are no foods with good or bad cholesterol in them.)

Now, you could have a total cholesterol reading of 220 and have nothing to worry about if it were made up of a lot of the good HDL cholesterol. On the other hand, you could have a so-called desirable reading of 180 but still be in trouble if a lot of it were made up of the bad LDL. Your total cholesterol number is not enough. You need to know what your cholesterol is made up of.

Your goal is to maximize the good HDL and to minimize the bad LDL. You want an HDL of at least 45 and an LDL of 100 or less. If you have other cardiovascular risk factors your LDL should be 70.

Another predictor of your future heart health is the ratio of your total cholesterol divided by your HDL. Your total cholesterol divided by your HDL should give you an answer of 3.5 or less when you put your own numbers in. For example, if you had a total cholesterol of 210 and an HDL of 70, then 210 divided by 70 is 3. At that result, you're less likely to have a problem when it comes to atherosclerosis, even though the total cholesterol in this case is above 200. Many people, unfortunately, don't have a ratio that gives them an answer of 3.5 or under.

Figure 10.1

WHAT'S *YOUR* RATIO?

$$\frac{\text{TOTAL CHOLESTEROL}}{\text{HDL}} = 3.5 \text{ or less}$$

The bottom line is that you need to know what your good HDL and bad LDL levels are. Period. If you don't know, find out.

What about triglycerides? The National Cholesterol Education Program has recommended that triglyceride blood levels not go above 200. But Dr. William Castelli, medical director of the Framingham Cardiovascular Institute, says anything above 150 is high. And recent research has shown that the number should not exceed 100 in people clearly at risk for heart disease.

Should you have your triglyceride level measured? It's usually done automatically when your physician orders blood work for your other cholesterol numbers. We now know that triglycerides *are* an independent, separate risk factor in and of themselves. They can help predict your future heart health. Yes, get yours measured.

And what should you do if you have high triglycerides? Other than drug therapy, many of the same steps that will improve your cholesterol reading will help decrease your triglycerides as well. Eating less fat (especially animal fat), getting rid of cigarettes, losing weight, and exercising will all help. Weight loss by itself is often all you need to get triglycerides down to where they should be. Eating less sugar and sugar-containing foods and avoiding alcohol can also help some people bring their triglyceride levels down. Surprisingly, the good omega-3 fats found in fish oils may also help bring down those triglyceride numbers.

> Many of the same steps that will improve your cholesterol reading will help decrease your triglycerides as well.

Should you take fish oil capsules? Some studies show that they can help. Fish oil capsules can have negative side effects for diabetics, however, if too many are taken. They can also slow down the time it takes for your blood to clot, which can be good or bad, depending on your particular health situation. Ask your physician to see if fish oil capsules are an option for you.

I suggest you eat more fish. What kind? Salmon and mackerel are among the richest sources of the omega-3 fats. You can avoid some of the recent concerns about contaminants, like PCB's, by eating less farmed salmon and choosing wild salmon instead. Ask for it. Canned Alaskan salmon is a safe bet too.

There's a relatively new kid on the block when it comes to heart disease risk. It's a substance found in the blood called *homocysteine*. The protein that you eat every day is made up of building blocks called amino acids. Among them is one called methionine. When a high protein intake and/or a deficiency of certain B vitamins in the diet causes methionine to build up, the methionine is converted into homocysteine, a dangerous substance.

Evidence is accumulating that high blood homocysteine levels may be associated with a higher risk for heart disease. Just like cholesterol, the higher your blood homocysteine level, the higher may be your risk of heart attack.

What do you do about it? Since there's more of the amino acid methionine in animal protein than in vegetable protein, you can cut down on your animal products. That's not a bad idea anyway, since most Americans are already getting twice the protein they need. High protein intake is often associated with a high fat intake too.

> Evidence is accumulating that high blood homocysteine levels may be associated with a higher risk for heart disease.

Another way you can help reduce your homocysteine level is to make sure you get an adequate intake of the B vitamins, especially vitamins B_6, B_{12}, and folic acid. *Whole* grain breads and cereals are great sources of folic acid and B_6. You can get folic acid from broccoli, beans, and spinach too. White flour, pasta, bread, white rice, and cornmeal are also now fortified with this important B vitamin. Additional sources of B_6 include potatoes, bananas, meat, and poultry.

With the exception of fortified cereals, B_{12} is only found in animal products like meat, fish, poultry, eggs, and dairy products. Strict vegetarians should probably choose a good breakfast cereal or take a vitamin B_{12} supplement. Of course, talk with your doctor and registered dietitian before starting any supplementation program.

Nonvegetarians can meet their needs for Vitamin B_{12} from foods like tuna, milk, yogurt, and, of course, fortified breakfast cereals. If you're regularly eating the other foods listed you're probably already getting what you need of B_6 and folic acid too.

A point of clarification. Even though high levels of blood homocysteine seem to be associated with a higher risk of heart disease, at this time we still don't have proof that lowering your homocysteine will prevent a heart attack. Logically it's probably a good guess, but the studies aren't in yet.

In the meantime, in my opinion, you should probably get your homocysteine levels measured when you're measuring your other cholesterol numbers. A reading of 5–9 micromoles per liter ($\mu mol/l$) is ideal. The steps necessary to reduce your homocysteine levels are good for overall health anyway. It won't hurt and it just might help.

Recent research has also discovered that cardiovascular disease can be related to an inflammation of the artery walls. That degree of inflammation can now be measured with a blood test that looks at levels of something called C-Reactive Protein. Ideal levels for the test, known as hs-CRP are less than 1mg/liter. It's been suggested that bacteria enter the blood and ultimately cause this inflammation. How do they get in? Periodontal dis-

> Learning about your cholesterol and other blood values is one of the best ways you can prevent the number-one killer.

Figure 10.2

KNOWING YOUR CHOLESTEROL NUMBERS

Total Cholesterol . . 150 mg/dl or less*

HDL . . . . At least 45
(The higher the better)

LDL . . . . 100 or less
(70 with heart disease)

Triglycerides . . . . Under 150
(Under 100 for those with other risk factors for heart disease)

Homocysteine . . . . 5 – 9 µmol/L

hs-C-Reactive Protein . . Under 1 mg/L

$\dfrac{\text{Total Cholesterol}}{\text{HDL}}$ . . . . . = 3.5 or less

Many variables can affect your results. For the most reliable readings, avoid strenuous exercise 24 hours before the blood test. Prolonged standing before your cholesterol test can potentially raise your cholesterol reading as much as 10 percent. Ideally, try to sit about 10 minutes or so before being tested. If you're being tested for LDL, triglycerides, homocysteine and/or hs-C-Reactive protein, you'll also need to refrain from all food and beverages except water for 12 hours before the test. Because readings can vary based on a woman's monthly cycle, women should schedule follow-up measurements at about the same time of month.

To be sure you've got an accurate reading, everyone should be retested anywhere from one to eight weeks after the first test and average the results. If you get a difference of over 30 points either way in your results, take a third test and average all three.

*The official recommendation is still "under 200." Contrary to earlier reports, a very low cholesterol number is not dangerous. Some cultures around the world that have very little heart disease have average cholesterol levels around only 100. The average worldwide cholesterol level is 165.

See Appendix I on page 247 for the official Canadian Recommended Blood Cholesterol Levels.

ease (bleeding gums) could be one explanation. It's estimated that about 80% of U.S. adults have some degree of periodontal disease. If you needed another reason to floss, this may just be it.

There's not an adult in this country who shouldn't know what his or her cholesterol numbers are. You are playing with fire if you don't know. Find out. It doesn't matter how good you feel. It doesn't matter if you're at your perfect weight. Nor does it matter if you've never smoked a cigarette. You need to know what's going on *inside* your arteries, and learning about your cholesterol and other blood values is one of the best ways you can prevent the number one killer.

11

Raising Your HDLs

L et's say your HDL level is too low. Keep in mind that if you have certain medical conditions like liver disease, gout, cystic fibrosis, or diabetes you can have a low HDL level even if you have a healthy lifestyle. If that's your situation, then medication to bring your HDLs up may help.

You can also have a decreased HDL level if you're currently taking medications like beta-blockers. Ask your physician if there are any alternatives that might still be effective without hurting your HDL level.

For most of us, however, a low HDL is the result of doing too many of the wrong things and not enough of the right things. So how can *you* get more of these good HDLs? Here are some suggestions that work.

CHOOSE GOOD PARENTS

To a large degree your "normal HDL" is determined by heredity. Some people are just born with a high HDL. But keep in mind that *genetics is your tendency, not your destiny*. If you tend to have a low amount of the good HDLs, there's a lot you can do to increase them.

PUT EXERCISE BACK INTO YOUR LIFESTYLE

You *must* have some kind of physical activity in your life. Choose some kind of aerobic exercise that you will do about three or four times a week. Get your heart rate going faster and break a sweat. However, recent research suggests that exercise needs to result in some loss of body fat in order to get a real boost in your HDL levels.

LOSE FAT

Obesity goes far beyond just how it looks. Being fat has an impact on practically every other aspect of your health. And people who have too much fat on their bodies—especially around their middle—can have less of the good HDL than leaner people. Take off the body fat, and your HDLs should go up.

EAT LESS FAT

Eating less fat can help you lose body fat, which, as we've said, should help increase your HDLs. On the other hand, when you decrease your dietary fat intake too much, your HDLs may actually go *down*. The recommended fat intakes we discuss in *Eating By The Book*, however, shouldn't hurt your HDLs. Also remember that it's your total cholesterol/HDL ratio, not just your HDL, that's also important. Eating less fat, especially animal fat, is still good advice.

Of the fat you do eat, try to make it olive, peanut, or canola oil. Recent research is suggesting that these monounsaturated fats are better than the polyunsaturates like corn, safflower, and soybean oil. While vegetable oils are, of course, better choices than animal fat, the monounsaturates are

probably better for your overall heart health. Equally important is that the mono's don't contribute to the inflammation
response like the poly's do. We're learning that inflammation
may aggravate all kinds of problems from arthritis to heart
disease. I use olive oil. It's got a nice long track record and the
cultures that use it generally enjoy better health than Americans do. If you don't like the strong flavor of olive oil, use the
"extra light." You can use it in any recipe in which you would
normally use vegetable oil. Besides, the Bible's been singing
the praises of olive oil for centuries (Deuteronomy 8:7–9; Exodus 30:22–25; Joshua 24:13; Nehemiah 9:25; Hosea 14:6).

GET OFF CIGARETTES

Anyone who smokes a pack a day has about twice the risk of
heart disease as a nonsmoker. Someone who smokes two
packs a day has three times the risk as a nonsmoker. On top
of all this, a smoker increases his or her risk of developing at
least eight different types of cancer and of having a stroke.

I know you've heard all this before. But, frankly, if you're
still smoking I don't know why you're reading a book on nutrition. You've got the cart before the horse. A lot of the health
problems that you're having or will have are due to the fact
that you're sucking that toxic smoke into your lungs 10, 20,
or 40 times a day. As a nutritionist I'd rather see you just continue to eat a lot of so-called junk food and put all your efforts
into getting rid of cigarettes.

If you're a cigarette smoker, I'd suggest you go to page 147
now and deal first with the number one preventable health
problem in this country. When you come back you will have
laid the foundation for successfully preventing a heart attack.

HAVE A DRINK?

Here's some good news. Research shows that moderate alcohol consumption is not only safe for most people, but it may
help prevent a heart attack.

Alcohol may also raise your good HDL. As usual, moderation is the important factor here. Keep in mind that a moderate level of alcohol consumption is no more than two drinks a day for a man or one drink a day for a woman. A "drink" is twelve ounces of beer, six ounces of wine, or 1½ ounces of hard liquor. While research shows that these consumption levels can provide some heart protection, amounts above that can cause real problems. Researchers have found that individuals who consume more than three drinks a day can raise their blood pressure–just what you don't want to do. Alcohol can also dramatically increase your triglyceride level. From a health standpoint, women are more sensitive to alcohol than men and are more likely to develop liver disease than their male counterparts. Consumption beyond one drink a day may increase breast cancer risk as well. Anyone with stomach ulcers or liver disease, or using certain medications needs to avoid alcohol completely. Ask your doctor.

If you don't drink, should you start? In a word, no. The potential risks from alcohol far outweigh any possible benefits. Keep in mind that even small amounts can cause problems for people with a history of alcohol abuse. Alcohol is a double-edged sword. It may possibly help your heart, and it can also potentially destroy your career, your marriage, and your life. There are so many other things you can do to reduce your risk of heart disease, you never need to drink alcohol. Having said that, if you do drink now and can keep it moderate as we've defined here, it's not going to hurt your heart, and it may help.

BE A WOMAN

If you're a woman you have a natural advantage of having a higher HDL than a man—at least up to the time of menopause. That's why you hardly ever hear of a woman having a heart attack in her 30s or 40s. After menopause, however, a woman starts to lose that advantage.

If you're a woman who's too young to be thinking about menopause yet, you may be taking birth control pills. "The pill" can actually lower the good HDL and raise the bad LDL. If you're on the pill, it's important that you know all of your cholesterol numbers. If you're doing everything right (in terms of food and exercise and not smoking), and your HDLs still aren't where they should be, you may want to talk with your physician about some other birth control alternatives.

CONSIDER NIACIN

This natural, very inexpensive B vitamin has been found to do wonders in increasing HDL levels. To be safe and effective, however, it requires a physician's supervision. See Chapter 18 on page 127 for more details on niacin and medications that can help raise your HDLs.

12

What About Eggs?

Basically, two substances will raise your total blood cholesterol number: cholesterol and fat. But the fat that you eat can raise your blood cholesterol *far more than* the cholesterol you eat. That sounds backward, but that's the way it is.

Your *liver* produces most of the cholesterol in your blood. And it can produce *a lot* of cholesterol when you eat a lot of animal fat, which, as you remember, we call saturated fat. Fat from animals can dramatically raise your blood cholesterol.

In one egg you only get one and a half grams of the bad saturated fat. So if you eat two eggs in the morning, that doesn't amount to much. In general, that would be fine. But keep in mind that eggs have a *lot* of cholesterol. In fact, one egg uses up almost your entire allowance of cholesterol for the day.

The current official recommendation is that it's okay to have up to four eggs yolks a week. I agree. You may personally be able to eat a lot more eggs than that with no problem, especially if you're eating a decreased-fat diet and you don't have high levels of LDL (the bad blood cholesterol) and/or triglycerides. The ability to handle dietary cholesterol can vary from person to person. But even if you're one of the lucky ones you can still overload the system with an excessive intake of cholesterol.

If you do want to cut down on eggs, remember that *all* of the fat and cholesterol are in the egg yolk. The egg white is basically pure protein and it's fat and cholesterol-free.

In many recipes you can substitute two egg whites for every whole egg called for. This works just fine in cakes, cookies, and pancakes as well as in many other recipes. Try using about four egg whites and only one yolk in an omelette, and put in a tablespoon of low-fat cottage cheese for every yolk that you leave out. The omelette tastes good and it looks good too—the one yolk still makes it look nice and yellow.

Throw the extra yolks down the drain. They won't clog your plumbing, but they might clog your arteries.

You don't have to be afraid of eggs—they're a good source of protein and other nutrients. As a dietitian, I'd much rather see people eat a few eggs a week and reduce their overall saturated fat intake than to see people completely avoid eggs but also not watch how much fat they take in.

> **I**f you do want to cut down on eggs, remember that *all* the fat and cholesterol are in the yolk. The egg white is basically pure protein and it's fat and cholesterol-free.

What about egg substitutes? They're fine. They're basically no more than egg whites with a little yellow food coloring and vegetable oil added. When you buy them you're paying for someone to take the egg yolk out for you. Egg substitutes are convenient, but you're paying extra for that convenience.

The bottom line on eggs is that you shouldn't eat more than four *yolks* a week. If you really need to bring your blood cholesterol levels down, even *that* may be too much. If you want to eat eggs, be sure your blood cholesterol numbers don't suffer as a result. Remember, too, that the eggs may not be the entire problem. It may be that the omelette is loaded with cheese and sausage and accompanied by an order of bacon, biscuits, and butter.

The bottom line on eggs is that you shouldn't eat more than four *yolks* a week.

13

Put the Salt Shaker Back on the Table!

Even though we're talking about cholesterol and its relation to your heart, it's important to point out another risk factor that can cause you problems even if your cholesterol numbers are perfect—high blood pressure.

The Source of Salt

Almost one-third of all adults in the United States have a problem with high blood pressure. By the time they're 65 years old, more than 60 percent of Americans have blood pressure that's too high. High blood pressure not only contributes to heart disease but also to stroke and kidney failure as well as to other problems.

Anything at or above 140/90 is considered actual high blood pressure, or by its official name, *hypertension*. A reading above 120/80 is designated as pre-hypertension. Your ideal goal is 120/80 or less. Now, hypertension doesn't necessarily mean that you're a tense or nervous person. You could be the most mellow, relaxed individual in the world and still have high blood pressure. You can't feel it, but you can do something about it.

Surprisingly, getting rid of your salt shaker is *not* the best way to fix the problem.

A good target intake for most Americans is 1,500-2,300 mg of sodium a day. Incidentally, for all practical purposes, you can use the words *salt* and *sodium* interchangeably. Table salt is actually the natural chemical called *sodium chloride*. If you're trying to cut back on your salt intake, look for the word *sodium* on the food label.

Your body only needs around 500 mg of sodium a day to function normally. That's the same thing as one-fourth of a teaspoon of salt. That's *all* you really require. The average consumption in this country is eight times that amount, at 4,000 mg—two teaspoons. You wouldn't think that little difference would matter. In fact, for some people it makes all the difference in the world!

> A good target intake for most Americans is around 2,000 mg of sodium a day.

Luckily, you don't have to go overboard and count every grain of salt to be healthy. Your body has the very nice ability to handle far more than 500 mg of sodium a day. That's why we're recommending a middle-ground intake of somewhere around 2,000 mg a day or less.

Let's say you want to cut down on your salt intake. What's the first thing to do? *Put the salt shaker back on the table!* What?? Yes, put it back where it belongs—back on the table right next to the pepper. Heresy? No, common sense.

Most people don't realize that 75 percent of the salt we take in every day comes, not from the salt shaker, not from what you add in cooking, but from the American supermarket.

Seventy-five percent of the salt we take in every day comes, not from the salt shaker, not from what you add in cooking, but from the American supermarket.

The majority of the salt we're taking in comes from processed, salt-added foods in our grocery store. And yet, in all due respect, the first thing many physicians do with a person who has been newly diagnosed with high blood pressure is to tell them to get rid of the salt shaker. The salt you add at the table, the salt you use in cooking, and the salt naturally found in foods only comes out to 25 percent of the salt you're taking in. *The salt shaker's not the problem!*

Using a salt substitute or getting rid of the salt shaker completely is like trying to put a raging fire out with a teaspoon of water. It helps, but not very much. If you're really serious about decreasing your daily intake of sodium, spend an hour in the supermarket.

Mmm, mmm, salty!

Let's look at a specific example. Consider a can of chicken noodle soup—the same product most of us grew up with and still use today. On the back of the can the sodium content is listed at 900 mg. Once again, a good healthy level of sodium for most of us, even those with high blood pressure, is around 2,000 mg a day.

Certainly 900 mg of sodium per serving is within the daily allowance. But you need to realize that the "soup people" assume you're only going to eat one-third of a can! I don't know about you, but I can consume the entire can without any problem. If one-third of a can has 900 mg of sodium, then you're actually getting 2,700 mg of sodium when you eat the whole thing. It's incredibly easy to consume far more than your daily sodium allowance even without using the salt shaker.

So don't necessarily restrict the salt shaker. Get educated about where the salt you're eating is *really* coming from.

Here's what you need to do. First of all, remember this: moderation, not perfection. Hardly anyone has a need to exclusively eat sodium-free foods. Thank goodness, since many of them taste terrible! Instead, start purchasing the no-salt-added, low-salt, and reduced-sodium products. While they may not taste as "good" as the regular high salt varieties, when you add a little salt from the salt shaker they'll be fine.

Read the label on the back of a regular 14.5 oz can of green beans. One national brand says it has 360 mg of sodium per serving. It also says one can serves 3.5 people! I don't think so. Maybe two people or one really hungry person.

> Get educated about where the salt you're eating is *really* coming from.

Nevertheless, at 360 mg of sodium per serving and 3.5 servings per can, there are 1,260 mg of sodium in one can of green beans. And they don't even taste salty! Most people will probably still add salt before they eat them.

Now look at the label on a can of no-salt-added green beans. One can still serves 3.5 people, but each serving only has 10 mg of sodium—making a total of 35 mg of sodium per can. Compare 35 mg to 1,260 mg. Now *that's* an improvement!

But you still have to do something about the rather bland taste. Here's an idea. Heat the green beans in a pan as you normally would. Add onions, spices, whatever you'd like for flavor, but don't add salt in cooking. Serve them as you've cooked them, and just before you eat, hit them with the salt shaker. The salt on the outside of the green beans will have a far greater positive impact on your taste buds than the salt that the food manufacturers added.

Since you probably won't add some 1,200 mg of sodium to your green beans, you're far better off by using the salt shaker.

Many people think that one of the saltiest items at McDonald's is the french fries. In fact, french fries are among the *lowest* salt items. McDonald's small fries only have 140 mg of sodium. That's a surprise since they taste so salty! The fries taste that way because the salt is

> French fries are among the *lowest* salt items at McDonalds.

on the outside of the food rather than cooked in. When the french fry hits your taste buds, you think you're getting a load of salt. McDonald's cookies—which don't taste salty at all—actually have more salt at 270 mg per serving! You don't really need to worry so much about foods that taste salty as you do about processed foods that have salt *in* them.

Not Just for Blood Pressure.

There are also several other potential benefits from reducing your sodium intake. Decreasing sodium may help prevent osteoporosis, the brittle-bone disease that affects so many women. We know that the higher your salt intake, the more calcium is found in your urine—and that that calcium is coming from your bones. A recent study showed that women who cut their salt consumption are also able to help prevent the loss of bone density normally seen at higher sodium intakes.

While adequate calcium intake is absolutely important for the prevention of osteoporosis, you may be able to get by

One of the most effective steps you can take to get your blood pressure down to a healthier level is to lose body fat.

with taking in less calcium if you also decrease your salt. Not only will your prospects for normal blood pressure be improved, but you'll have stronger bones as an added bonus.

Several studies suggest that cutting down on salt may also help those who suffer with asthma symptoms.

What if you do cut down on your salt consumption and you still can't budge your blood pressure? A diet with lots of fruits, vegetables, and low-fat dairy foods every day seems to help. But one of the most effective steps you can take to get your blood pressure down to a healthier level is to lose body fat. By eating less fat and putting regular moderate physical activity into your lifestyle, you not only lose body fat but you also strengthen your heart, which, in turn, can help to lower your blood pressure.

Increasing your calcium intake may also help reduce blood pressure. If you drink alcohol, reducing your intake to no more than two drinks per day for a man or one drink per day for a woman can also help.

Caffeine may also raise your blood pressure, so try decaf and other noncaffeinated drinks instead.

Smoking cigarettes damages and constricts your blood vessels. If you smoke and want to control your blood pressure, get rid of those cigarettes.

It may be possible to avoid high blood pressure medication if you make some minor diet and lifestyle changes. Nevertheless, if you've tried all of these options and your blood pressure is still too high, then your physician may indeed prescribe medication. If so, take the medicine faithfully.

As part of the treatment, they will often give you a diuretic to help your body get rid of excess water. Diuretics usually work very well, but they can decrease the amount of potassium in your body at the same time. To help make up for this loss, eat more foods that contain a good amount of potassium such as baked or boiled potatoes, bananas, fat free milk, cantaloupes, raisins, and oranges. However, unless your physician says otherwise, do not take potassium supplements on your own. Potassium supplements can be lethal at a consumption level of just five times the recommended daily intake.

Once again, you can't "feel" high blood pressure. If you do need to take medication, you may need to take it for the rest of your life or until you get rid of the cause or until your physician tells you otherwise—regardless of how you feel. Some side effects such as fatigue and impotence are possible with medication. Nevertheless, even with side effects, as undesirable as these symptoms might be, you're still far better off than suffering from the death or disability that high blood pressure can bring. Keep in mind that a healthy lifestyle can also mean you'll need a smaller dose of medication, and that can mean fewer side effects.

> High blood pressure is serious; work with your physician in controlling it.

High blood pressure is serious; work with your physician in controlling it.

You may have recently heard that the official recommendation that *all* Americans restrict their salt intake may have been a little overenthusiastic. I agree. The fact is that most Americans' blood pressure will *not* go down—or up—based on their salt intake. It's estimated that only a third of us are salt sensitive. Most of us won't see much of a change in our blood pressure regardless of how much salt we consume. Nevertheless, a lot of people, especially those who already have high blood pressure, *will* benefit from cutting down on their daily sodium consumption. Additionally, we have no way of testing to determine if *you* as an individual are salt sensitive. Therefore, even though many could handle more, the official recommendation of around 2,000 mg of sodium per day is still a good idea.

If you have high blood pressure, remember that even a little drop in your blood pressure numbers can mean a big improvement in your long-term health. Even though you're not considered to have high blood pressure until you're at 140/90 or more, a good goal is 120/80 or less.

> Even a little drop in your blood pressure numbers can mean a big improvement in your long-term health.

More than half of all Americans develop high blood pressure as they grow older. You can decrease your chances of that ever happening if you're more conservative in your salt intake today.

Figure 13.1

WOW! THAT'S GOT A LOT OF SALT!

Your daily sodium goal should be somewhere between 1,500–2,300 mg. If you have high blood pressure, your physician may suggest even less. These few examples demonstrate just how easy it is to get a lot of sodium— even if you don't use the salt shaker.

FOOD	Quantity	Sodium (mg)
Chicken noodle soup	1 can	2,700
Hungry-Man Chicken TV Dinner	1 serving	1,940
Tomato sauce, canned	1 cup	1,480
Spaghetti sauce	1 cup	1,280
Soy sauce	1 tbsp	1,260
Big Mac	1 serving	1,050
Whopper	1 serving	1,020
Arby's Regular Roast Beef Sandwich	1 serving	950
Tomato juice	1 cup	860
Cottage cheese	1 cup	840
Chicken Pot Pie	1 serving	780
Dill Pickle	3 oz.	720
Frozen Pizza—12"	1/4 pizza	680
Gravy, canned	1/2 cup	620
Hot Dog	1 serving	610

14

Don't Worry, Be Happy!

Stress is perception. It's not the event, the boss, or the job that's stressful—it's your reaction to it.

Someone could have the exact same high-pressure job as you do and not experience stress. Why? You may fear the loss of your job, whereas the other person may know he could find another one.

You may fear that a stock market crash would ruin you, and the other person may know that even if it did crash, he still has the ability to continue to generate an income.

> Do not be anxious about anything, but in everything . . . present your requests to God. And the peace of God . . . will guard your hearts and mind in Christ Jesus.
> *Philippians 4:6–7*

> A cheerful heart is good medicine.
> *Proverbs 17:22*

While stress may be all in your head, its results often show up in your health. Too much stress can increase your risk for high blood pressure, high blood cholesterol, heart disease, and cancer. It can also decrease your body's ability to fight infection. A study at Harvard found that men who experienced high anxiety had up to a six-times higher chance of sudden cardiac death.

Why are we anxious? Why are we stressed? Often it's self-induced. Our desire for "things" often stretches us beyond our means. A bigger home, a bigger boat, and a bigger debt can indeed make any threat to your paycheck seem to be monumental. And yet what does God say? Matthew 6:25–33 tells us:

> Therefore I tell you, do not worry about your life, what you will eat or drink; or about your body, what you will wear. Is not life more important than food, and the body more important than clothes? Look at the birds of the air; they do not sow or reap or store away in barns, and yet your heavenly Father feeds them. Are you not much more valuable than they? Who of you by worrying can add a single hour to his life?
>
> And why do you worry about clothes? See how the lilies of the field grow. They do not labor or spin. Yet I tell you that not even Solomon in all his splendor was dressed like one of these. If that is how God clothes the grass of the field, which is here today and tomorrow is thrown into the fire, will he not much more clothe you, O you of little faith? So do not worry, saying, "What shall we eat?" or "What shall we drink?" or "What shall we wear?" For the pagans run after all these things, and your heavenly Father knows that you need them. But seek first his kingdom and his

righteousness, and all these things will be given to you as well. Therefore do not worry about tomorrow, for tomorrow will worry about itself. Each day has enough trouble of its own.

It's not that we are to be oblivious to the needs of our families and ourselves, it's just that God asks us to trust Him and not worry about it. If you're seeking first the kingdom of God and His righteousness, you probably won't be trying to "keep up with the Joneses."

You may have heard that Type A people have been found to be at higher risk for heart attacks. They're the kind of people who are always trying to do four or five things at once, are always on the go, and may even finish your sentence for you if you're not talking fast enough for them.

We've now learned that type A personalities suffer from no more health problems than do the more relaxed type

> **A** man of knowledge uses words with restraint, a man of understanding is even-tempered.
> *Proverbs 17:27*

B people—unless they exhibit one particular trait called anger. Go-getters who have explosive bouts of anger have heart attacks.

A recent study found that "the men who were the most calm and thoughtful in their speech were the least likely to die during the study." The risk comes not from being on the go so much as it does from not being able to let it go. James 1:19–20 tells us:

> My dear brothers, take note of this: Everyone should be quick to listen, slow to speak and slow to become angry, for man's anger does not bring about the righteous life that God desires.

If we are truly acting by Jesus' example and being servants to our fellow man, and if we get rid of our pride, there should be very few things that we allow to get us angry. Not only is stress management good for your spiritual health, it's good for your physical health as well.

Better a patient man than a warrior, a man who controls his temper than one who takes a city.
Proverbs 16:32

15

What's a Woman to Do?

Heart disease is the number one killer of women in this country. You don't hear much about that fact because we know more about heart disease in men than we do in women. Most of the studies that have looked at the problem have used men because heart disease tends to show up earlier in males.

But did you know that more women now die from heart disease every year than men? It's true! And when a woman has a heart attack she is more likely to die from it than her male counterpart.

On the positive side, women have a built-in factor that often protects them from heart disease for a while–estrogen. This naturally occurring hormone that a woman produces in her body helps decrease her risk for heart problems, everything else being equal.

For example, consider a married couple who eat the same food and who are the same age and who are both at ideal weight. In general, the woman has a smaller chance of a heart attack than he does. That's true during her entire life, up to the time of menopause. After a woman's estrogen levels decrease, however, she starts to play by the same rules as her husband always has.

Heart disease is the #1 killer of women in this country. More women now die from heart disease every year than men.

After menopause, the older a woman gets, the greater her risk of getting heart disease. From ages 45 to 64 only one out of every seven women has this problem. But after age 65, the risk increases to one out of two! The majority of women in the United States still have cholesterol levels *above* the official desirable level of 200. Make no mistake about it. As a woman your number one health threat is not breast cancer; it's heart disease.

So what's a woman to do? All the lifestyle changes that help men reduce their risk also help women. Eat less fat, especially animal fat. Stay off cigarettes. Control high blood pressure. Exercise. Maintain your blood cholesterol numbers at a desirable level.

Keep in mind that studies show that a woman's cholesterol readings may fluctuate based on what part of her menstrual cycle she's in. So if you're trying to improve your blood cholesterol readings and want to monitor your progress, be sure you have your blood drawn at about the same part of your cycle every time you have it measured.

Since *pre*menopausal women are protected from heart disease by naturally produced estrogen, should *post*-menopausal women take hormones in pill form? The recent Women's Health Initiative study has clarified our understanding about hormone replacement therapy (that is, estrogen and progestin taken together). Hormone replacement therapy does, in fact, decrease osteoporosis risk. It also decreases your chance of getting colorectal cancer. However, as was suspected, breast cancer risk is increased. The major surprise has been the discovery that it *raises*, not lowers, your chance of heart disease. This is the opposite of what was believed for years. For those women who just take estrogen by itself, the research has shown a decrease in osteoporosis risk but also an increase risk of stroke.

Here's what you need to know. Estrogen or the estrogen/progestin combination is now only recommended for those women who are having severe menopausal symptoms. The research has shown no danger from taking these for about four years or less which is all many women need to get though menopause. The recommendation is to take the lowest dose for the shortest amount of time. The risk of health problems start to rise when they're taken for longer periods, however. If you're on hormones now, ask your physician about slowly taking you off. If you're taking them for the prevention or treatment of osteoporosis ask about the medications called Fosamax, Evista, Boniva, and Forteo. They're relatively new medicines that have been shown to decrease your osteoporosis risk without the negative side effects of traditional hormone replacement therapy.

> Find a physician who realizes that heart disease is as real of a risk to a woman as it is to a man.

16

Margarine or Butter?

A while back there was a great deal of talk about palm, palm kernel, and coconut oil and how they were probably not very good for you. Let's do a quick review.

A Trip to the Tropics

Fat comes in two varieties: saturated and unsaturated. Saturated fat is the kind you find in animal products like butter and meat. Unsaturated fat, like corn oil and olive oil, comes from plant sources. For the most part, saturated fats raise your blood cholesterol and unsaturated fats may help lower it.

There are some vegetable fats, however, that go around acting like animals! Palm oil, palm kernel oil, and coconut oil obviously all come from plants and therefore should be unsaturated. But they are the *exception*. Even though they come from plants they're saturated fats. We don't know why that is, that's just the way God designed them.

This presented a problem for consumers. Food manufacturers who used these three oils could still label their products as using "100% vegetable oil." Most people (correctly) thought that vegetable/plant oils were a healthier choice than animal fat and therefore (incorrectly) bought those products. Since they are saturated fats, the palm, palm kernel, and coconut vegetable oils actually had the potential to raise a person's blood cholesterol once they ate the product. The food manufacturers were technically telling the truth by identifying vegetable oil on the front label, but they weren't telling the whole truth.

> There are some vegetable fats that go around acting like animals!

The public finally caught on and, in one of the few instances where consumers flexed their financial muscle, they got most of the manufacturers to take out these so-called tropical oils. Manufacturers now use other vegetable oils like canola, soybean, corn, and others. That's certainly an improvement over before, but there's more to the story.

Today many foods like chips, crackers, cookies, and commercially baked items no longer contain coconut oil, palm oil, or palm kernel oil. But now, for example, instead of seeing soybean oil listed on the label, you'll see something called "partially hydrogenated soybean oil" or "partially hydrogenated canola oil." What's that all about?

When manufacturers make baked goods, they often get a better product if they use a solid fat (like shortening) rather than a liquid fat (like vegetable oil). If you've ever made a pie crust you know that the solid fat gives a much more desirable flaky crust than does the liquid oil. Not only is the commercially baked product better looking, but the product lasts longer on the store shelf too.

Another name for solid fat is saturated fat. An easy rule to remember is that if it's solid at room temperature it's saturated and that if it's liquid at room temperature it's unsaturated. Lard is solid at room temperature, so it's saturated. Corn oil is liquid, so it's unsaturated.

Why do I bring all this up? When food manufacturers stopped using saturated fats like palm oil, palm kernel oil, and coconut oil, they had to find replacements, such as canola oil, corn oil, and soybean oil. The baked goods made with these unsaturated fats, however, didn't have as good of a taste, texture, and shelf life as the baked goods made with saturated fats.

So what's a food manufacturer supposed to do? The public won't buy his products if he uses saturated fats like lard or palm oil or coconut oil. If he switches to a better oil like canola or corn, his product doesn't turn out as well. He's concerned that the consumer won't buy it that way either.

Yankee Ingenuity

The manufacturers came up with a rather unique idea. They found that when an unsaturated oil is exposed to hydrogen, it acts more like a saturated fat. Thus you can *hydrogenate* an unsaturated fat to give you a better product and yet still claim on the label that you're using one of the good unsaturated oils.

When an oil is *partially hydrogenated*, the oil will be partially saturated. That means that the partially hydrogenated oil will now act more like a saturated fat. But it's still not as bad for you as if they had used an actual saturated fat like butter, lard, palm oil, or coconut oil.

So what's the point? When you artificially partially hydrogenate an oil you change its normal chemical structure from something called *cis*, to a rather unusual structure called *trans*. In very simple terms you bend the fat molecule. Now don't be confused by all this chemistry. When a food manufacturer partially hydrogenates an oil, he partially changes the structure of that oil into something that isn't usually found in that food.

Here's the crux of the issue. Some research is now showing that these partially hydrogenated oils that are used today are probably no better than the saturated fats they replaced!

Recent studies have shown that, when compared to people eating the regular nonhydrogenated oils, people eating these trans fats (the partially hydrogenated fats) raised both their total blood cholesterol and their bad LDL cholesterol just as much as if they had consumed the regular bad saturated fats. So even though, theoretically, these partially hydrogenated fats still should be "less bad" than the saturated fats they replaced, the research is indicating that they are, in fact, no bargain either.

Is Butter Better?

Finally, we get to the margarine vs butter issue. As you probably know, margarine was basically created as a replacement for butter. Since margarine is made from vegetable oil, it should be less bad than the saturated animal fat called butter. As a result, for the last 30 years or so, margarine has been promoted as the spread of choice.

But research is now showing that margarine has the potential to raise your blood cholesterol too! Based on what we've been talking about, that shouldn't be much of a surprise. Because you probably don't want to pour liquid corn oil on your toast in the morning, the food manufacturers add hydrogen to the unsaturated oil and partially hydrogenate it, in the process making it more solid and more saturated.

Now it looks more like the butter it's supposed to replace, and you can spread what used to be corn oil on your toast in the morning and everybody's happy. However, since it's partially hydrogenated, it now contains the trans fats.

Today it's hard to avoid these partially hydrogenated fats. Just look at the food labels in your kitchen cabinet right now and you'll see them listed. They're in everything from cookies and crackers to coffee cakes, margarine, breaded-and-fried chicken and fish, snack foods like potato chips, and even in fast-food french fries. Do you need to avoid these foods? No. Do you need to eat less of them? Probably yes.

So what should you do about all of this? Should you go back to butter? No. Should you start baking with lard again? Certainly not. Butter and lard are saturated animal fats and we *know* that they definitely don't do you any good.

Keep in mind: *The good news about all of this trans, partially hydrogenated oil situation is that it's not that much of an issue if you're not eating much fat.* And once again the lesson, as we've said from the beginning, is to *eat less fat.*

If you're not eating much fat, then it really doesn't matter so much if that little bit you're eating is saturated or unsaturated or partially hydrogenated. The less total fat you're eating, the less important is this issue. Hopefully you're starting to eat more of the reduced fat and fat free products available in the supermarket anyway. When you do, in addition to reducing your risk of heart disease, cancer, and obesity, one more bonus is that you *don't have to worry* about this partially hydrogenated trans-fat issue.

> **P**artially hydrogenated oils used today are probably no better than the saturated fats they replaced!

Here's more good news. Some food manufacturers are no longer hydrogenating the oils in some of their products. They'll even say "no trans fats" right on the front of the package. Not only is the fat in many of these products often low, but it's also not hydrogenated. I like that.

What should you put on your toast in the morning? Butter or margarine? Neither. Use jelly or honey. Both of these are fat free. And even though they're sugar based, sugar isn't nearly the health threat to you that fat is. I'm not defending sugar; it's empty calories and it doesn't do anybody any good. But fat is the bigger problem.

The bottom line between butter and margarine? Go with margarine. Even though it has the trans fatty acids from hydrogenation, there's not enough of them to raise your blood cholesterol as much as all the saturated fat in butter does. A tablespoon of butter has about 11 grams of total fat, 7 of which are saturated. A tablespoon of margarine also has 11 grams of total fat but only has 2 grams of saturated fat and about 2 grams of trans fat; the rest is unsaturated fat. The total of the "bad" fats in margarine still doesn't equal what you get in butter. On top of that, butter has cholesterol, but regular margarine doesn't.

Here are a few more suggestions. First, choose the tub or liquid margarine, which has less trans fat, instead of the more solid stick forms. Second, read the label. The total trans fat grams per serving is now listed on most labels. The less, the better. Finally, look for new products like trans fat free margarine. As more and more food manufacturers start producing more of these products, this issue may become even less and less important. As for now, try finding products made without hydrogenated or partially hydrogenated fat.

> The bottom line between butter and margarine? Go with margarine.

Butter or margarine? Margarine.

17

What About
My Children?

Should you be concerned about your children's cholesterol? Autopsies performed on American children reveal
that they have fatty streaks in their arteries as early as age
nine! Heart disease may show up when you're sixty or sev-
enty but it may start as early as the first decade of life.

Lack of activity and the weight gain that comes as a result
can raise blood cholesterol levels in children. The number of
overweight children in this country has risen tremendously
in the last twenty years. This could mean future problems
with diabetes, high blood pressure, and heart disease for these
children.

Today's kids aren't necessarily eating more calories, but
they are a lot less active. Only about a third of U.S. schools
still offer any kind of physical education classes.

During childhood, our main goal is to provide adequate
nutrition, not to prevent disease. However, the evidence is

becoming clear that atherosclerosis and heart disease often have their beginning stages in childhood.

But keep in mind that we don't want to reduce fat so much that the child doesn't get enough calories to grow. At the same time, however, we *do* want to begin to show that

> Atherosclerosis and heart disease often have their beginning stages in childhood.

child that the low-fat foods that the rest of the family is eating *can* taste good. If you help a child who's three or four years old get used to lower-fat foods, by the time that child is 13 or 14 you won't have much trouble. On the other hand, if you wait to introduce lower-fat, healthier foods until the teenage years, you may have a real problem on your hands.

A recent federal advisory panel suggested that all children over the age of two start eating lower-fat, lower-cholesterol foods. This does not apply to infants, however. Below age two, children still need more fat for growth and nerve development. But for all other children, eating less fat and cholesterol is now the goal.

The panel also suggested that children who come from families with a history of heart disease or high blood cholesterol levels should also have their blood cholesterol levels checked. That means that about one out of every four children should get a blood cholesterol test now. Any child who has diabetes or is severely overweight should also be tested.

If a teen or preteen smokes, he is already increasing his risk of cholesterol problems. Should you have them tested? No, you should lock them up in a room until they're about 21 and come to their senses!

Every day 3,000 kids start smoking. One-third of them will eventually die from that decision. One of the best things you can do for a youngster is to make sure he never starts smoking. We know that if a young person can make it to about age 21 without cigarettes, odds are he never will smoke.

Should we test all children for cholesterol? No, according to the official recommendation. Not all children with high cholesterol levels become adults with high cholesterol levels. However, many *do*. In fact, studies show that children with high cholesterol levels are about three times more likely to have elevated levels when they become adults. If it were my child, I'd want to know if there was a potential problem so I could take some appropriate conservative action now rather than wait 15 or 20 years. I would have them tested.

What are the blood cholesterol levels we'd like to see in a child? For total cholesterol, the official guideline is anything between 120–230. But if there's a family history of heart disease, the numbers are more conservative. Talk to your physician and registered dietitian to see if some moderate changes in the child's diet won't improve their readings.

Helpful Hints

What improvements can you make in the foods that a child will eat? For starters, you can bake or broil meats instead of frying them. At fast-food restaurants the skinless chicken sandwiches are a good choice as well. Many children, and adults too, find the frozen yogurts not only acceptable but actually often just as tasty as the higher fat ice creams. Also, go to fat free or 1% milk rather than whole or 2% and try the lower-fat or fat free cheeses when you make a sandwich. Pretzels and popcorn are good low-fat snacks too, but with microwave popcorn be sure to get the kind that is reduced in fat.

While we're on the topic of children let's also briefly mention weight control. Twenty percent of all American children are overweight, and this number has been rising over the past 20 years. The average child sees 5,000 food commercials every year, and most are for high-fat and high-sugar foods.

The most important point regarding weight management in children is to avoid putting them on a very low calorie diet. Children need calories to continue to grow and mature to their full genetic potential. If a child is overweight we don't want to restrict calories so much that he ends up short in height because he didn't have enough energy to grow on.

In dealing with a child who's overweight, try to help him maintain his weight and let him grow into it as he grows taller. If a child is 20 pounds overweight now and you can help keep him there, over the course of a couple of years as he grows taller he'll probably end up where he should be.

How do you help a child maintain his weight? In many ways you should use the same methods you use for yourself; watch his fat and sugar intake and encourage him to get more exercise. As we've said, only about a third of all children get any kind of formal exercise. A little less TV, a little more activity, and less fat and sugar intake will work best for most children who have a weight problem.

Do we emphasize specific weight guidelines for children? No. Overemphasis in this area may be contributing to the rising rates of anorexia and bulimia, and the preoccupation with weight that we see in so many adolescents today, especially in teenage girls. Nevertheless, the risk of

> Twenty percent of all American children are overweight.

becoming an overweight adult is about twice as high for someone who was overweight as a child as compared to someone who was normal weight. A child's chances for adult obesity are increased when he continues his excess weight into adolescence.

Incidentally, if you want to prevent obesity in your child's future, take some pounds off yourself. A study in the *New England Journal of Medicine* found that what parents weigh can affect the *future* weight of their children. Normal-weight children up to age 10 have more than twice the risk of adult obesity if their parents are obese. But being an overweight child contributes to the problem too. In this study an obese 15- to 17-year-old had a 54 percent higher risk of adult obesity if the parents were normal weight, but a 73 percent higher risk if they were obese themselves.

The most immediate concerns with childhood obesity are the psychological and social factors that accompany the problem. From a very early age, overweight children are often ostracized and ridiculed. This can have a serious and long-term effect on the self-image of children and adolescents. *Prevention* of excess weight gain will go a long way to help assure long-term psychological and physical health in children.

Prevention of excess weight gain will go a long way to help assure long-term psychological and physical health in children.

18

Just Take a Pill

What if you've tried everything we've talked about for six months and you still haven't had any luck getting your cholesterol down? You've cut your fat intake, you exercise three or four times a week, you got rid of the cigarettes, you've lost weight and, after all that, your cholesterol numbers are still not where they need to be.

Not too long ago you would have been out of luck. Now, fortunately, we have a variety of medications that *will* get the job done. But, as always, we want to use medicine as a last resort only after we've tried all other improvements in lifestyle and diet first.

As in everything we've been talking about, it's important that you work with your physician. Realize that there is no one magic pill that works for everyone and that you and your physician may have to try several different brands to find the one that works best for you. But if you've honestly been doing everything right for at least six months and your numbers are not heading down, then you and your physician need to consider which medications might help.

If your cholesterol numbers are not where they need to be (see page 85) and your physician doesn't seem all that concerned about it, find another physician! Heart disease is serious business. If you just wait for something to go wrong, it most likely will. Don't get yourself in a position where you have to depend on medical technology to keep you from dying. Instead, take an *active* role in keeping the good health God has given you.

> Take an *active* role in keeping the good health God has given you.

Here's what's available today to assist you in your efforts to lower your blood cholesterol numbers:

Psyllium

One of the least expensive and easiest ways to initially lower your numbers is to try a product like Metamucil or Konsyl. There are a number of brands available, and even the less expensive house brands work as long as they contain the ingredient called psyllium.

Psyllium comes from a grain most commonly grown in India and acts not only as a laxative but also nicely normalizes bowel habits in general. This fiber is totally natural, and you cannot develop a dependency upon it.

One additional benefit is that psyllium is the kind of fiber that may also lower blood cholesterol levels by 5 percent, 10 percent, or even more. This is where I would start if I were you—simply follow the directions on the container. You might want to start with a rounded teaspoon every day. It's also very important that you drink adequate water with this product. Psyllium is safe and effective for the vast majority of people. However, some individuals can have a sensitivity to psyllium. As always, of course, ask your physician.

Aspirin

If you reach the point where you and your physician are considering medication to lower your cholesterol numbers, you might also consider taking an aspirin. Research has shown that taking a single 81 mg baby aspirin tablet every day may have the same or even greater effect on preventing a heart attack than does lowering your cholesterol numbers with medication. Ask your physician.

Although the aspirin won't actually lower your cholesterol numbers, it nevertheless seems to decrease your risk of having a heart attack. Research has also shown that aspirin can help prevent the reoccurrence of a heart attack or stroke if you've had one already.

How does it work? Aspirin seems to decrease your chances of having a blood clot. Since blood clots often are the reason for a heart attack or stroke, aspirin reduces your risk.

If you're at risk for a heart attack or stroke, you may want to actually carry aspirin in your pocket or purse. Studies have shown that taking an aspirin as soon as heart attack or stroke symptoms appear can significantly increase your chances of survival. The American Heart Association recommends that in this situation you take a full dose 325 mg tablet. It's important, however, to get that aspirin into your blood system almost immediately. Don't just swallow it. Chew it first and then swallow. It may not be very tasty, but it could save your life.

Aspirin is an inexpensive over-the-counter medicine that can keep you alive. As if that weren't enough, aspirin has also been shown to decrease your risk of colon cancer, cataracts, diabetic eye problems, and maybe even breast cancer. It may also help prevent some senility problems often associated with aging. Experts believe that a large portion of decreased mental functioning seen in the elderly is due to blood clots that form in the brain. If you or someone you care for is starting to show symptoms of mental deterioration, aspirin therapy may be a good idea.

Today, most aspirin is used for the prevention of heart disease, not for headaches. Does that mean *you* should take aspirin for your heart health? If you're a man over 50 with one risk factor or a woman who has gone through menopause with two risk factors, you probably *will* benefit from taking aspirin. Those risk factors include being physically inactive, obese, diabetic, or being a smoker. You're considered at risk, too, if you have high blood cholesterol or high blood pressure, or if heart disease or stroke runs in your family. That covers *a lot* of people.

Aspirin doesn't agree with everyone, however. If you have stomach ulcers, kidney or liver disease, you're already using anti-clotting drugs like Coumadin, or you're allergic to aspirin, you're probably better off to avoid it. Nevertheless, it's safe to say that many people who would benefit from daily conservative aspirin therapy still aren't taking advantage of it.

It's also important to remember that we're not talking about taking just *any* pain-relief medicine. It needs to be aspirin. Acetaminophen (Tylenol) and Ibuprofen (Advil) don't have the same protective effects.

As always, your doctor knows your health history and status better than anyone. It's always appropriate to start slowly, to watch for side effects, and to make sure the medication fits into your lifestyle.

Niacin

You may have heard about the effectiveness of the B vitamin niacin on reducing cholesterol levels. Niacin can lower the bad LDL cholesterol, it can increase the good HDL, and it can also reduce triglycerides. You can't ask for much more than that!

The amount of niacin that you need to take to achieve these results, however, is far greater than the amount you need merely for good health. In fact, at these amounts niacin is considered a medication, not just a vitamin. Nevertheless, it can be extremely effective and is very inexpensive.

Niacin comes in two forms—nicotinic acid and niaci-namide. Only nicotinic acid lowers cholesterol. Be sure to check the label of what you're taking.

Many people complain of a temporary flushing and itching of the skin after taking the vitamin. To help minimize this effect, take the niacin with a meal rather than on an empty stomach. You can also alleviate some of this problem by taking an aspirin 30 minutes before you take the niacin. If your physician has you on aspirin anyway, the combination may help. Finally, don't start with a full dosage of niacin right away. A lot of people have more success when they slowly increase the dosage of niacin over the course of several weeks.

At the higher dosage we're talking about, you need to be under the supervision of your physician. I can't emphasize that strongly enough. No one should take niacin to reduce blood cholesterol without working closely with his doctor. There is always a potential for problems with the liver, blood sugar, gout, and especially intestinal discomfort at these high levels.

You probably want to steer completely clear of the time-release form of niacin since some research indicates that it may lead to liver problems and other negative side effects. Now don't let all of this keep you from trying niacin. Work with your physician. Many people take it quite comfortably.

Niacin can help get your cholesterol numbers back to good healthy levels, and it's a lot less expensive than the other medications. Additionally, the combination of niacin with other cholesterol medications can have a greater effect than either therapy alone.

Bile-Acid Sequestrants

The first place many physicians started in the past was with this category that included medications called cholestyramine, colestipol, and colesevalam, known by such brand names of Questran, Prevalite, Colestid, and Welchol. These medications lower the bad LDLs.

Cholestyramine and colestipol attach themselves to bile acids in your intestine, thus causing them to be excreted rather than reabsorbed back into your body. That's important because the bile acids that your body produces are made from cholesterol. So when your body has to replace the bile acids that get lost, it uses up some of your cholesterol to do so. As a result, your blood cholesterol goes down.

> We want to use medications as a last resort only after we've tried all other improvements in lifestyle and diet first.

When taking these medications, be sure to take sufficient fluids to avoid constipation. Unfortunately, these medications may increase triglycerides, so if you already have high triglyceride levels you should avoid them. These medications may also interfere with the absorption of other drugs you're taking. As a result, fewer prescriptions are being written for this category of medication.

Fibric Acid Derivatives

Gemfibrozil (Lopid), Fenofibrate (Tricor), and Clofibrate (Atromid-S) are alternatives to the bile-acid sequesterants. These seem to work especially well for those people who have high triglyceride levels. Gemfibrozil and Fenofibrate bring down the bad LDL moderately and appear to increase the good HDL at the same time. There is, however, a question regarding the safety of this drug category as it relates to increased cancer risk.

Statins

Without a doubt, the most exciting relatively new category we have in our battle against high blood cholesterol levels has a fancy name of HMG-CoA reductase inhibitors; also called the "statins." These include simvastatin (Zocor), lovastatin (Mevacor), atorvastatin (Lipitor), pravastatin (Pravachol), fluvastatin (Lescol), and rosuvastatin (Crestor).

Altocor is an extended release form of Mevacor that slowly enters the blood throughout the day, rather than all at once like the other statins. It will probably save you money too since it's cheaper than even the generics.

The statins work by reducing the amount of cholesterol the liver produces. Of all the medications available, the statins are the most effective at lowering the bad LDL cholesterol. And they have very few, if any, side effects for most people. In fact, in two major studies, less than one percent of the participants reported problems.

A study of over 6,000 men with high cholesterol levels who had never suffered a heart attack found that the group who took Pravachol eventually had one-third fewer heart attacks than the group taking a placebo pill. In another study of over 4,000 men, no increase in death from cancer was found in those men who took a statin, and they had a total decrease in death rate of 30 percent.

> **M**edications help control the cholesterol situation but do not cure it.

This is exciting! We now have the ability to decrease your risk *of even a first heart attack* without the potential of causing other problems. Although atorvastatin seems to lower the bad LDL and triglycerides even better than the rest, in general all the statin forms seem to have about the same cholesterol-lowering effect. There seem to be few, if any, problems with short-term side effects. We still don't know if there will be any long-term negative consequences but they've now been safely used for a number of years on millions of people. Today, the statins often are the drug of choice.

There's not one perfect medication out there for everyone. While the statins look good, they may not be best for *you*. One type of drug may help one person, but you might benefit more from a different type. It all depends on you and your particular cholesterol profile. Some people even take more than one medication at the same time for the best results. Your physician, of course, is the best judge of that.

The bottom line on medication is that options are now available for you if you can't improve your numbers to healthy levels without it. The general consensus is that if diet and exercise don't work well enough, you should consider starting with the statins. These medicines are an exciting breakthrough. It appears that you can now not only use the statins to treat but actually to prevent the progression of heart disease without causing some of the serious side effects of the other medication categories.

Keep in mind that the statins are not magic pills. You will still need to eat significantly less fat and increase your physical activity. You will still need to be regularly monitored by your physician for any potential side effects. And most likely you will still have to stay on the medication for the rest of your life.

Zetia (ezetimibe) is another medication that can be taken alone or in combination with a statin. While the statins work on cholesterol production in the liver, Zetia works in your intestine by actually limiting the amount of cholesterol that gets absorbed. It's less effective than the statins so you probably won't take it alone. However, if the statins don't lower your bad LDL cholesterol enough, combining them with Zetia can be more effective than even doubling the dose of a statin. Zetia is also better tolerated than the bile-acid sequestrants that doctors often prescribe when statins alone don't get the job done.

The cholesterol medication called Vytorin is a combination of Zetia and the statin Zocor.

Studies show that unhealthy cholesterol numbers will return if you stop drug therapy. These medications help control the cholesterol situation but do not cure it. You and your physician can certainly experiment as time goes on. If you're being successful at reducing your cholesterol numbers, the two of you may want to decrease the dosage of your particular medication. You can then monitor your numbers to see if your body will still give you the good results without the quantity of medication that may have been necessary up to that point.

If you've tried everything else and you've been unsuccessful, don't overlook this incredible opportunity to help improve not only the quantity but the quality of your life.

PART II

ACTION STEPS
FOR HEART DISEASE PREVENTION

1. **Stop smoking now!** Use a patch, chew the gum, take the pill, do whatever it takes. The very best thing you can do for your health is to get tobacco products out of your life!

2. **Find out what your cholesterol numbers are.** A finger prick that only gives you total cholesterol doesn't tell you much. Get your total cholesterol, HDL, LDL, triglycerides, homocysteine, and hs-C-Reactive Protein levels measured. Be sure to get retested within eight weeks to make sure you have accurate readings.

3. **Take off excess body fat.** Assuming you don't smoke, your number one health priority is to slowly take excess fat off your body. The best way to do that is to eat less fat and sugar and put physical activity into your lifestyle.

4. **Eat less fat—especially animal fat!** Over time, replace whole dairy products with low-fat and fat free products. Research and personal experience indicates that if you'll stick with it for six months, you'll actually start to *like* lower-fat products. Switch from butter to reduced fat or fat free soft tub margarine. Better yet, put jelly or honey on your toast in the morning—they're both fat free.

5. **Put physical activity into your lifestyle.** Even if you already have heart disease, physical activity can help your body's blood vessels build collateral circulation around narrowed arteries. As a result, even if an artery becomes blocked, there may still be enough blood flow to your

heart muscle to prevent what otherwise might be a full-blown heart attack or even death.

6. **Get your high blood pressure under control.** Simply losing excess body fat will bring the blood pressure of many adults back to normal. If you're on medication now, you may need to decrease the dosage after you lose fat. Work with your physician.

7. **Put the salt shaker back on the table and get educated about where the salt is *really* coming from!** If your physician disagrees, take him to a grocery store!

8. **Teach your child to eat lower-fat foods.** Remember, it's much easier to raise a child on lower-fat foods than it is to change the dietary habits of a teenager.

9. **If your blood cholesterol numbers don't start coming down to where they should be in six months or so, ask your physician about medication.** High cholesterol numbers are *serious*! Don't wait for something to go wrong. Prevent a heart attack before it happens!

Additional Resources
for Heart Disease Information

The American Heart Association
General information about the association and chapters. Reliable information source for health care providers and patients.

    7272 Greenville Ave.
    Dallas, TX 75231
    1-800-242-8721
    www.americanheart.org

The Mended Hearts, Inc.
Over 250 local chapters around the U.S. and Canada providing support to heart disease patients and their families. Affiliated with the American Heart Association.

    7272 Greenville Ave.
    Dallas, TX 75231
    214-706-1442
    www.mendedhearts.org

Heart Information Network
Up-to-date educational information on heart disease, prevention, and treatment.

    www.heartinfo.org

National Heart, Lung, and Blood Institute
Reliable information on the prevention and treatment of high blood pressure.

    P.O. Box 30105
    Bethesda, MD 20824
    301-592-8573
    www.nhlbi.nih.gov

PART
III

CANCER: PREVENTION IS THE BEST MEDICINE

19

The Dreaded Diagnosis

Fifteen hundred people died today from cancer. About 1,000 of them didn't have to. We already know enough to *prevent two-thirds* of all cancers. What we don't know yet is how to get people to take responsibility for their own health.

Of the half million or so people in the United States who die each year from cancer, most of them could still be alive and well if they had stopped smoking and improved the quality of the food they ate. Everyone knows smoking causes cancer. Most people still don't know that a poor diet causes about *the same number* of cancer cases.

No technology or medicine can *make* you stop smoking. The decision must come from within you. No device or drug will lift you off the couch or

> Fifteen hundred people died today from cancer. About 1,000 of them didn't have to.

make you eat broccoli. The desire to live long enough to see
your grandchildren grow up—and the effort to do something
about it—must come from you alone. Regardless of any new
breakthroughs in cancer research, the information already
known can help most of us beat cancer before it ever starts.

As deadly as heart disease is, many people fear a diagnosis of cancer even more. When I worked at a hospital I'd hear
physicians and nurses talking about *C-A*. It took me a while
to figure out they were discussing patients with CAncer. Even
some health professionals are uncom-
fortable saying the word. The fear is
justified.

> One out
> of every four
> deaths in
> this country
> is caused
> by cancer.

Cancer causes one out of every
four deaths in this country and is the
second biggest killer. Cancer causes
pain that can linger for months and
even years.

Many people mistakenly believe
that heart disease is a rather quick way
to go. In fact, today most people who
have a heart attack *do* survive. More often than not, though,
they never return to the same quality of life they had before
their heart attack. Additionally, the same dangerous process
that often brings on quick heart attacks also causes strokes,
and the effects of a stroke can last the rest of your lifetime.

Neither cancer nor heart disease is a good way to go, and
neither is better than the other.

Slow but steady progress is being made on those cancers
that aren't directly related to lifestyle decisions. In the 1930s,
an average cancer patient had only a 20 percent chance of
being alive in five years. In the 1940s it was up to 25 percent,
and by the 1960s it was 30 percent. Today the average five-
year survival rate is 40 percent.

You may not be impressed with this kind of progress if
you're the one with cancer, but the news is far better than it

appears. The average five-year survival rates are so modest because they include lung cancer. If you exclude that particular disease, the rate is much better.

In the last 30 years, deaths from colorectal cancer are down 9 percent in men and down 31 percent in women. Liver cancer is down 13 percent in men and down 45 percent in women, and stomach cancer is down about 60 percent in both men and women. Bladder cancer and Hodgkin's disease are also both down, and the cancer death rate in children is down a reassuring 62 percent!

Early detection before the cancer spreads has a lot to do with your chance of beating this killer. Your odds of preventing cancer, however, are far, far greater than your chances of getting cured from it.

Tables 19.1 and 19.2 (pages 144–145) show clearly that the main cancer threats to women are lung, breast, and colorectal cancers. For men the cancer threats are lung, prostate, and colorectal. Breast cancer gets so much publicity when, in fact, lung cancer kills far more women every year. Perhaps in addition to encouraging women to get regular mammograms, we should put even more effort into keeping their teenage

> Your odds of preventing cancer are far, far greater than your chances of getting cured from it.

daughters from lighting up their first cigarette. If current trends continue, the incredible number of new teenage female smokers will become the future victims of lung cancer as adults.

Figure 19.1

YEARLY CANCER DEATHS
BY SITE—FEMALES

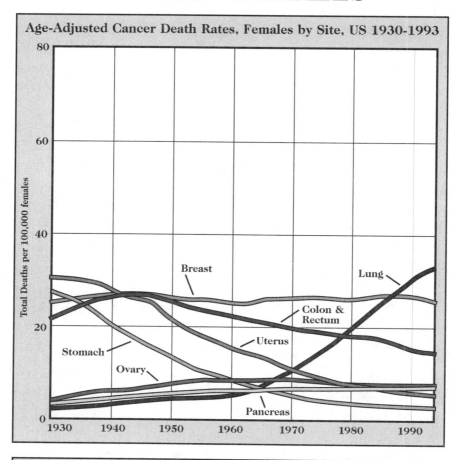

Age-Adjusted Cancer Death Rates, Females by Site, US 1930-1993

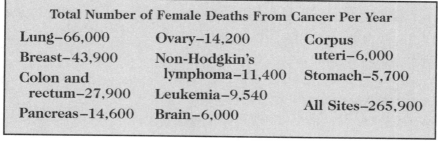

Total Number of Female Deaths From Cancer Per Year

Lung–66,000   Ovary–14,200   Corpus
Breast–43,900   Non-Hodgkin's   uteri–6,000
Colon and   lymphoma–11,400   Stomach–5,700
  rectum–27,900   Leukemia–9,540
Pancreas–14,600   Brain–6,000   All Sites–265,900

Figure 19.2

YEARLY CANCER DEATHS
BY SITE—MALES

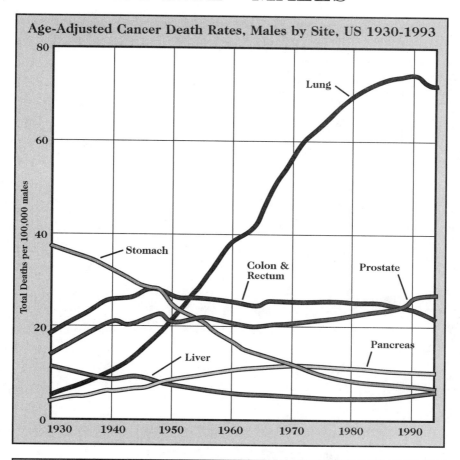

Age-Adjusted Cancer Death Rates, Males by Site, US 1930-1993

Total Number of Male Deaths From Cancer Per Year

Lung–94,400	Non-Hodgkin's lymphoma–12,400	Urinary bladder–7,800
Prostate–41,800	Leukemia–11,770	Liver–7,500
Colon and rectum–27,000	Esophagus–8,700	All Sites–294,100
Pancreas–13,500	Stomach–8,300	

20

The Marlboro
Man Is Dead

Stop smoking now. Stop smoking now. Stop smoking now.
Period.

Is that clear enough? Cigarette smoke contains over
4,000 different chemicals. Many of them have been proven to
cause cancer. I'm amazed at the number of cigarette smokers
who are worried about preservatives and additives in their
food. The chemicals in their cigarette smoke will kill them
long before the chemicals in their food will.

The number one cause of preventable health problems in
our society today is the fact that people set dried leaves on
fire and inhale the smoke deep into their lungs. How could
any right-thinking person do such a thing? If your neighbor
raked the leaves in his yard this fall, set them on fire, and
came out of his house 20 to 40 times just to suck in the
smoke, you might call the authorities! And yet that's exactly
what cigarette smoking is.

Oh, smoking cigarettes may be more socially acceptable

than smoking yard leaves, but it's becoming less acceptable every year. It's true that not *all* lung cancer is caused by cigarettes—only a mere 87 percent! The rest is caused by such factors as air pollution, second-hand smoke, asbestos, and radiation.

Even though more people get breast, prostate, and colon cancer every year, lung cancer still *kills* more American men and women than the others, simply because it's so deadly once you get it. On the average, only 13 percent of those with this cancer are still alive five years after the diagnosis. This year about 160,000 Americans will die from lung cancer. A lot of them will die simply because as teenagers they thought smoking was cool.

If you won't quit smoking cigarettes for your own health, do it for your kids or grandchildren. One study says that parents who smoke contribute to the deaths of about 6,000 children in the U.S. each year. Of that, 2,800 deaths can be attributed to the low birth weight of children born to mothers who smoked during pregnancy. Another 2,000 children die from sudden infant death syndrome caused by second-hand smoke, and 1,100 die from respiratory infections.

> Parents need to think long and hard about whether that cigarette is really worth the price.

Another study indicated that boys whose mother smoked during pregnancy were four times more likely to demonstrate antisocial behavior such as stealing and vandalism when they got older. And parents who smoke caused another 5 million(!) children to suffer from asthma and ear infections.

We don't own these little ones. God has only loaned them to us for a short while. Parents need to think long and hard about whether that cigarette is really worth the price.

Most people who develop lung cancer are over 50 years of age and have a long history of smoking cigarettes. Of course that doesn't mean you have nothing to worry about if you're under 50. You don't suddenly "get" lung cancer. It takes a number of years for the cancer to show up.

On the positive side, it's never too late to quit smoking, even if you're over 50. You can cut your risk for lung cancer in half within 10 years of stopping. Even better news, your risk of heart disease will be cut in half within one year of getting off of cigarettes. And even if you don't add a single day of life from stopping, you will definitely improve the *quality* of your years.

> I t's *never* too late to quit smoking.

And here's some more good news. The rate of lung cancer in American men has actually started going down in the last several years.

Because of new technology? No. Because of better surgical techniques or drugs? No. Because men seem to finally be getting the message. It's not a dramatic drop, but it is a drop in the rates that up to this point kept going up and up every year.

Unfortunately, earlier in this century it became socially acceptable for women to start smoking in public. Now many of those same women are paying the price for a lifetime of cigarette dependence. That's why the number of women with lung cancer is growing faster than from any other form of the disease.

What are the warning signs? *Don't wait for warning signs!* The presence of chest pain, continual bouts of pneumonia or bronchitis, and a persistent cough or bloody sputum are warning signs you never want to see.

You say you're worried about gaining weight if you stop smoking? The fact is that many people *will* gain five to 10 pounds as a result of getting cigarettes out of their life. While you may not like the way the extra weight looks, you'd have to gain an extra *100 pounds* to equal the risk as if you had continued to smoke two packs of cigarettes a day.

Excess weight gain is certainly not good for your health, but cigarettes are far worse. Besides, if you can finally, successfully, once-and-for-all get cigarettes out of your life, then losing weight is easy by comparison. If you're able to kick the nicotine addiction, you *can* take excess fat off your body. You've already learned how in the earlier chapters.

Make no mistake, smoking cigarettes *is* an addiction. The drug, which is legal, is called nicotine. It nevertheless is still a drug, and telling a smoker to "just stop smoking" is in many ways like telling a heroin addict to "just stop shooting."

For most people, getting off cigarettes is not just a matter of will power. Once your body gets used to nicotine it will fight you if you try to get off of it. There are lots of reasons to keep smoking, but there's no excuse. Today we have so many ways, including medications, to kick the habit once and for all that even if you've tried before you need to keep on trying.

Most successful former smokers finally succeeded on their *third or fourth serious try.* Many were dismal failures on their first couple of attempts, so keep on trying! You may be closer to success than you realize.

> There are lots of reasons to keep smoking, but there's no excuse.

Ask your doctor about the medication called *Zyban*. It doesn't contain any nicotine, and yet it's the most effective medication now available to permanently get you off cigarettes. It's often combined with "the patch" or another nicotine source for an even improved rate of success. Zyban is available by prescription only, so ask your doctor about the best approach for your particular situation.

You didn't come into this world smoking, and you lived many years of your young life without ever having a cigarette.

You got along just fine without them. Your body does *not* have a *requirement* for nicotine; it has an *addiction* to nicotine. Getting off of cigarettes will be terribly uncomfortable for a while, but if literally millions and millions of other people have done it, so can you.

21

Mammography Mania

Here's what you've been told. In the 1940s a woman's chance of having breast cancer sometime in her lifetime was 1 in 20. By the 1970s it was up to 1 in 13. Today it's 1 in 8. That doesn't sound too encouraging. But here's the *good* news you may not yet have heard about breast cancer. The odds of getting breast cancer during your *lifetime* have gone up not because there's an epidemic of breast cancer but because women are living longer and being diagnosed earlier.

Since breast cancer shows up primarily in older women, the longer you live the greater your chance of getting it. Don't let that news damper your enthusiasm for longevity. From that perspective, the only option of reducing your lifetime risk of breast cancer is to die early. That's not such a good choice.

Since mammography finds breast cancer earlier than self-examination, and since the baby boom generation has expanded the actual number of women in those susceptible years, a greater number of women are being diagnosed with the disease. But, *there is no epidemic of breast cancer!*

Even though the *incidence* of breast cancer has been steadily growing in the past, even that now seems to have leveled off. Only about 1 woman in every 1,000 will be diagnosed with breast cancer this year. From Figure 21.1 on page 156 you can see that, in fact, *death* rates from breast cancer are basically unchanged since the 1930s! In fact they've now come down by more than 5 percent in the last several years.

It's good that women are being educated about the need to monitor for breast cancer, but shouldn't we be putting *at least* that much effort and attention in preventing *lung* cancer as well?

Here are some numbers to consider. By age 40, a woman's risk of getting breast cancer in the next ten years is only 1 in 65. If you live to be 50, your odds have increased to 1 in 41. By age 60, you have a 1 in 29 chance, and not until you're in your 90's is your risk 1 in 8. This should be *very good news* for those of you under 90!

Even though breast cancer is probably the disease women fear the most, that anxiety is misplaced. A woman's risk of getting heart disease after age 65 is 1 in 2! The reality is that *most women will never get breast cancer.* And even if a woman does get it, the average five-year survival rate today is a very reassuring 83 percent because of early detection and mammography.

> The reality is that most women will never get breast cancer.

The theme of *Eating By The Book* is prevention. So even though the news is good about your risk of actually ever getting breast cancer, let's see if we can make your odds even better. If you can avoid or minimize the following risk factors, you'll go a long way toward preventing the problem.

As we've said, the risk rises with age. There's not much

you can do about your age, but you can relax a little bit until you get to be about 90. If you began your period earlier than most girls or had a later-than-average menopause, your risk for breast cancer is increased. The longer lifetime exposure to the estrogen your body naturally produces may contribute to the formation of the cancer cells.

Surprisingly, women with a higher risk for breast cancer are also better educated, and/or have never had children. Having your children after age 30, making more money than the average woman, and being obese are also all risk factors. Now we can't explain all of these; we just observe that that's the case.

So should you avoid education? Make less money? Of course not. You should, however, sincerely consider working on reducing your risk in those areas that make sense.

> Death rates from breast cancer are basically unchanged since the 1930s!

We used to think that a high fat diet increased your risk for breast cancer, but the most recent research seems to put the blame more specifically on saturated fat.

Research also indicates that even as little as one drink of alcohol a day may increase your risk of breast cancer as well. So even though you may have heard some good news about having a glass of wine to reduce your risk of heart disease, you may not want to do so if that same glass of wine puts you at a higher risk for breast cancer. If you don't drink now, don't start.

Self-exams and visits to that physician are the first line of defense for early detection of breast cancer. Annual mammograms are highly suggested for women over 40 and recommended for women over 50.

What are the warning signs of breast cancer? Any skin irritation, pain, or discharge from the breast. Also any lump, swelling, thickening, or dimpling. Remember, *you* are your very best health advocate. If you're concerned about something and your physician isn't, get another opinion!

Figure 21.1

WHAT ARE YOUR REAL ODDS?

You've heard that one in eight women will get breast cancer. But that's true only if you live to be 95! Here are the odds for everyone else:

80 years old	1 in 16
70 years old	1 in 24
60 years old	1 in 29
50 years old	1 in 41
40 years old	1 in 65
30 years old	1 in 233
20 years old	1 in 2,500

22

Do You Take This Man . . .?

The *Journal of the National Cancer Institute* recently reported, "A sexually transmitted virus is the major cause of cervical cancer among women worldwide." It seems logical, therefore, the fewer sexual partners a woman and a man have in their lifetime, the lower her chances of contracting this deadly disease.

A number of studies have found that a woman is much more likely to get cervical cancer if her husband has sex outside of marriage. Hebrews 13:4 says, "Marriage should be honored by all, and the marriage bed kept pure, for God will judge the adulterer and all the sexually immoral." There is less

> **A number of studies have found that a woman is much more likely to get cervical cancer if her husband has sex outside of marriage.**

chance of cervical cancer if a woman and her husband honor God's Word.

In Genesis 2:18 God declared that "It is not good for the man to be alone. I will make a helper suitable for him." Studies now indicate that people, especially men, who are married have better health than those who are divorced, widowed or single.

Even beyond the formality of marriage, being with other people is just plain good for you. You do better as an individual when you're part of something bigger than just your own little world, whether that something is your church, your club, or your family and your friends. The Bible teaches how important companionship is in Ecclesiastes 4:8–12:

> There was a man all alone; he had neither son nor brother. There was no end to his toil, yet his eyes were not content with his wealth. "For whom am I toiling," he asked, "and why am I depriving myself of enjoyment?" This too is meaningless—a miserable business!
>
> Two are better than one, because they have a good return for their work: If one falls down, his friend can help him up. But pity the man who falls and has no one to help him up! Also, if two lie down together, they will keep warm. But how can one keep warm alone? Though one may be overpowered, two can defend themselves. A cord of three strands is not quickly broken.

It appears that God created us to be in relationships with one another. Scripture says in Hebrews 10:25, "Let us not give up meeting together, as some are in the habit of doing, but let us encourage one another."

A University of Michigan study found that older men who did not remain active and had less social contact were more likely to die during the study than men who participated in volunteer activity and generally kept themselves connected with other people.

A number of studies are now showing a higher divorce rate for people who live together before marriage than for people who don't. One study found that women who remain virgins until marriage were less likely to divorce. In addition, live-in boyfriends were found to be more likely than were married men to physically abuse their partners.

> Studies are now showing a higher divorce rate for people who live together before marriage than for people who don't.

Regular church attendance has also been shown to dramatically decrease a couple's chance of divorce. In fact, couples who report no religious affiliation at all appear to have the highest risk for early divorce. Even when separation does occur, the chances for reconciliation are higher among those who attend church regularly.

God's purpose is not to keep us from enjoying life. His goal is not to take away your pleasure or keep you from having fun. God isn't against sex. After all, it was His idea! But He does know that the most intimate relationship between a man and a woman will work best within the protection of marriage. He knows what works in this world and what doesn't. He knows the intricacies of human relationships because, after all, He's the one who created the intricacies of human relationships. It just makes sense to follow what He says.

God gives most of us years and years of life to grow in our trust and obedience of Him. Along the way He gives us daily, real-life opportunities to develop that obedience. All we have to do is follow what He says. Obedience will give us a life that is protected and blessed.

23

What's That Glove For, Doctor?

Every day more than 100 American men die from prostate cancer, and its incidence is increasing every year. Men don't like to talk about it, and they certainly don't like to get tested for it. An exam by your physician is the first line of defense in early detection.

But a digital rectal exam is not high on most men's favorite-things-to-do list, and less than half the men who need the exam are actually having it done.

Yes, it's embarrassing.

Yes, it's uncomfortable.

Nevertheless, you should be doing it every year after the age of 40. It's not that bad. Do it anyway.

> Every day more than 100 American men die from prostate cancer.

If you won't do it for yourself, do it for your children and grandchildren. Do it so your wife doesn't lose her husband.

The prostate is a gland about the size of a walnut that produces the seminal fluid that carries sperm. It surrounds the base of the urethral tube, which carries urine from the bladder out of the body. An infected, enlarged, or cancerous prostate can inhibit the urethra and cause painful and frequent urination, bloody urine, and pain in the thighs, pelvis, and back.

The amount of fat a man eats may influence whether he will get this cancer. Men in Japan, who have a lower fat intake, have less prostate cancer than American men. Eating a lot of fat can cause a man's body to produce more testosterone. More testosterone can, in turn, cause the prostate to enlarge and, if already present, promote the growth of cancer cells. This may be one reason why black men, who have slightly higher testosterone levels, have a 37 percent higher prostate cancer rate than white men.

Almost half of all prostate cancers are detected when it's too late.

A digital rectal exam will catch about 60 percent of prostate cancers. But if you have a PSA (prostate specific antigen) blood test, the detection rate goes up to 70 percent. The PSA test isn't the final word by itself, however. Combining both tests, digital and PSA, is the way to go from age 50 on.

Almost half of all prostate cancers are detected when it's too late. This isn't because the cancer spreads so fast. It's because men are too slow in making an appointment.

24

This Won't Hurt a Bit!

In the 1950s and 1960s almost all baby boys born in the U.S. were circumcised. Then in 1975 the American Academy of Pediatrics issued a statement that said that there were "no valid medical indications for circumcision in the neonatal period."

Circumcision was seen primarily as a procedure that was based on religious tradition, and the general recommendation was that newborn boys need not be put through the discomfort of the procedure.

Today, only about 65 percent of baby boys in the U.S. are circumsized. However, since that statement in the 1970's a study of over 400,000 newborn boys found that those who were not circumcised had an 11-fold increase in the incidence of urinary tract infections. While rare, cancer of the penis has been found to occur basically only in those men who are uncircumcised or circumcised after infancy. Recent evidence is now also suggesting that circumcised males also are less likely to acquire certain sexually transmitted diseases, including AIDS. So in 1989 the American Academy of Pediatrics clarified their position and said that while the procedure did have risks, it also had potential benefits and advantages.

> Today the majority of health professionals in this country once again endorse circumcision.

But hold on. They've changed their minds *again!* In 1999 that same group said that the benefits were not significant enough to recommend circumcision as a routine procedure. Then in 2000, the American Medical Association followed suit and said that while there are potential medical benefits, the research wasn't strong enough to recommend routine circumcision.

But *God* recommends routine circumcision! Genesis 17:9–11 says:

> Then God said to Abraham, "As for you, you must keep my covenant, you and your descendants after you for the generations to come. This is my covenant with you and your descendants after you, the covenant you are to keep: Every male among you shall be circumcised. You are to undergo circumcision, and it will be the sign of the covenant between me and you."

Paul says in 1 Corinthians 7:19 that "Circumcision is nothing and uncircumcision is nothing." Today we know for a fact that the procedure has definite physical benefits. Paul didn't know that 2,000 years ago. He was simply talking from a *spiritual* standpoint. And, of course, we agree with that. Circumcision does not sanctify you; circumcision does not save your soul. Ceremonial circumcision is an outward sign that the baby boy is a child of God. From this perspective, circumcision is certainly just as appropriate today as it was when God originally commanded it.

We've now learned, however, that there are also real physical benefits to be received *above and beyond* those that would be expected in the spiritual realm.

Vitamin K is used by the body to help clot blood. Without it, even a minor cut could become a serious situation. Yet you don't need to worry about eating vitamin K since it's actually produced by bacteria in your intestines! These tiny organisms live off a little of the food in your gut, and, in exchange, they produce the vitamin K that your body then absorbs.

Babies are not born with these so-called friendly bacteria, and so they don't produce vitamin K. Once they're born, however, simple human contact allows the bacteria to be introduced and vitamin K production to begin. It takes about *seven days* for the body to have enough vitamin K to start to be effective in blood clotting.

God's Word says in Genesis 17:12: "For the generations to come every male among you who is eight days old must be circumcised." And in Leviticus 12:3: "On the eighth day the boy is to be circumcised."

> Long before science figured out what was going on, the Bible showed God's people the right way.

God's Word says that baby boys are to be brought for circumcision at the very time that their bodies will for the first time be able to deal with the procedure. Even a day or two earlier could prove to be very dangerous.

Today, to be on the safe side, most babies receive injections of the vitamin when they're born. Nevertheless, how wonderful that long before science figured out what was going on, the Bible showed God's people the right way.

25

All We Are Saying Is Give Peas a Chance

After lung cancer, the most common cancer is found in the colon. Fortunately colon cancer is not nearly so deadly. If detected early before it spreads, the average five-year survival rate is 61 percent. While your risk for getting many cancers is influenced by what you eat, it's even more true for colon and rectal cancers.

Fat and fiber appear to be the key elements in prevention. The most dangerous dietary habit appears to be a diet high in fat and low in roughage. In fact, many studies indicate that

After lung cancer, the most common cancer is found in the colon.

eating a low-fat diet over your lifetime can cut your risk of colon cancer in half.

In the U.S.—where we still eat way too much fat—our risk of colon cancer is about three times higher than in Japan, where they eat much less fat than we do. Since the introduction of fast foods and Westernized diets into the Japanese culture, however, their colon cancer risk has gone up dramatically over what it was twenty years ago.

> To reduce your risk of cancer, eat more fruits, vegetables, beans, and *whole* grain breads and cereals.

Animal fat, as opposed to vegetable fat like olive oil and corn oil, appears to be especially dangerous. The "Nurses Health Study" found that those who ate the most animal fat had almost twice the risk of developing colon cancer as those who ate the least. Remember, our biggest sources of animal fat are fatty red meats and *whole* dairy products. And even though we've been talking throughout *Eating By The Book* about making moderate changes in your diet, it appears that the maximum allowable amount of fat intake to prevent colon cancer is probably lower than the maximum amount of fat allowed just to prevent heart disease. A conservative intake of animal fat is always a good idea.

A diet high in fiber will go a long way in reducing your risk as well. It's been estimated that you can cut your chances of colon cancer by about 40 percent if you're getting 25–30 grams of fiber a day. Most of us currently only get around 10 grams a day. There are several different kinds of fiber. To get a good variety, be sure you eat both whole grain products and fruits and vegetables. You need three to five servings of vegetables, two to four servings of fruits, and at least six servings of whole grains *every day*. Peas, beans, and lentils are great sources of fiber too.

Roughage helps take some of the risk out of a high-fat diet. However, this doesn't mean that if you're getting plenty of fiber you can ignore your fat intake.

When you eat a diet with lots of fat, the liver secretes bile into the intestine to help digest it. The more fat consumed, the more bile released. Unfortunately, bile acids and their by-products are similar in structure to known carcinogens. Fiber seems to dilute the impact of bile acids and so potentially decreases their danger. The bottom line for the prevention of colon cancer is to eat less fat and eat more fiber.

Good nutrition can help reduce your overall cancer risk too. Eating more foods rich in beta-carotene like cantaloupe, carrots, sweet potatoes, broccoli, and spinach will help. Vitamin C foods are also effective and include citrus fruits, strawberries, and tomatoes.

> Cruciferous vegetables like broccoli and cauliflower get their name because their flowers form a cross (or crucifix).

Avoiding or really cutting back on alcohol consumption and limiting your intake of salt-cured, smoked, and nitrite-cured foods are also good ideas.

Proverbs 23:2 says, "Put a knife to your throat if you are given to gluttony." There's evidence now that a high-calorie diet also significantly increases a person's risk for colon cancer. Obesity in your midsection seems to be risky as well.

We know from animal studies that if you restrict calories in those that already have cancer, you can prevent the tumors from growing and can stop new ones from developing. Cancer cells, like all cells, need energy to grow. With excessively high calorie intake, you may simply be stoking the fire of cancer growth.

If you're over 40, an annual digital rectal exam and stool blood test are recommended. Once you reach age 50, a sigmoidoscopy every three to five years will help you detect any cancer in the early stages.

What are the warning signs of colon and rectal cancer? Bloody stools, change in your bowel habits, and rectal bleeding. While these symptoms don't necessarily mean cancer, they should get you to a physician *quickly* to make sure. If colon cancer is detected early, your chances of survival are *very* good. Don't wait.

ACTION STEPS
FOR CANCER PREVENTION

1. **Get cigarettes and all tobacco products out of your life.** Get help. Your addiction to nicotine is no stronger than it was for the millions and millions of people who are now successful former smokers.

2. **Whatever it takes, see to it that the young people in your life *never start* smoking or using tobacco products.** A lifetime of good health is among the best legacies you'll ever leave for your children and grandchildren.

3. **Keep in mind that poor diet and nutrition accounts for just as many cancer deaths as do cigarettes.** For good quality nutrition see Chapters 26-27 on pages 179-194 and "The Rules to the Game" on page 195. The bottom line on nutrition and cancer prevention is to increase fiber and decrease fat.

4. **If you're a woman, be sure to do regular breast self-exams and, after age 40, get periodic mammograms.**

5. **If you're a man over 40, have your doctor check your prostate as part of your regular medical checkups.** After age 50, you should also have the PSA blood test done as well.

6. **If you're a man or woman over 40, get tested for colon and rectal cancer.** Wouldn't you rather go through a little discomfort now than experience the pain of surgery—or worse—later?

7. **Get educated.** Contact the resources on pages 175-176 for the information that's most important for you and your family.

Figure 25.1

EAT MORE ROUGHAGE!

Remember: An adult's eventual goal is about thirty grams of fiber per day. But, give yourself a couple of months to reach that level.

EXCELLENT SOURCES
(7 OR MORE GRAMS)

Raspberries . . . . 1 cup
All Bran Cereal . . . . 1/3 cup
Fiber One Cereal . . . . 1/2 cup
Oat Flakes Cereal . . . . 2 oz.
Butter beans . . . . 1/2 cup
Great Northern beans . . . . 1/2 cup
Kidney beans . . . . 1/2 cup
Navy beans . . . . 1/2 cup
Broccoli, cooked . . . . 1 stalk
Health Valley Veg. Chili w/beans . . . . 4 oz.
Prunes . . . . 1 cup
Split peas . . . . 1/2 cup
Health Valley Almond & Date Oat Bran Muffin . . . . 1 muffin
Post Raisin Bran . . . . 1 cup
Health Valley Real Italian Minestrone Soup . . . . .1 cup

VERY GOOD SOURCES
(5–6 GRAMS)

Blackberries . . . . 1/2 cup
Brussels sprouts . . . . 1 cup
Turnips . . . . 1/2 cup
Black beans . . . . 1/2 cup
Black-eyed peas . . . . 1/2 cup
Pinto beans . . . . 1/2 cup
Spinach, cooked . . . . 1/2 cup
Lentils . . . . 1/2 cup
Progresso Healthy Classics Lentil Soup . . . . 1 cup
Spoon-Size Shredded Wheat . . . . 1 cup
100% Whole Grain Wheat Chex . . . . 3/4 cup
Pita, whole wheat . . . . 1 pita
Almonds . . . . 1/4 cup

VERY GOOD SOURCES (Continued)

Quaker Plus Fiber Hot Cereal . . . . 1 pkg.
Raisins, seedless . . . . 1 cup
Red beans . . . . 1/2 cup

GOOD SOURCES
(2–4 GRAMS)

Oatmeal . . . . 1/3 cup
Popcorn . . . . 3 cups
Pumpernickel bread . . . . 1 slice
Rye bread . . . . 1 slice
Sweet potato . . . . 1/3 cup
Apples 1
Nectarines . . . . 1 med.
Apricots 4
Figs, dried 2
Grits . . . . 1 cup
Oranges 1
Pears 1
Plums 2
Corn, cooked . . . . 1/2 cup
Prunes, dried . . . . 4 med.
Strawberries . . . . 1 cup
Beets . . . . 1/2 cup
Lima beans . . . . 1/2 cup
Banana . . . . 1 med.
Brown rice . . . . 2/3 cup
Peanut butter . . . . 2 tbsp
Peaches . . . . 1 med.
String beans . . . . 1/2 cup
Peas . . . . 1 cup
Wild rice . . . . 1 cup
Winter squash . . . . 1/2 cup
Quaker Quick Oats . . . . 1 cup
Aunt Jemima Buckwheat Pancake Mix . . . . 4 pancakes
Baked potato w/skin 1
Tortilla, whole wheat 1
Nabisco Wheat 'n' Bran Triscuits 7
Wonder 100% Whole Wheat Bread . . . . 1 slice

Figure 25.2

WHAT CAUSES CANCER DEATHS?

Here are estimates of the extent to which various factors contribute to the incidence of cancer deaths in the United States. You can see that it doesn't make much sense to move to the country to avoid big city pollutants (2 percent) if you're still going to eat a lot of fat in your diet (30 percent) when you get there. The point of these numbers is not to predict your particular risk; rather it's to show how unnecessary it is to worry about radiation from electric power lines if you still smoke cigarettes.

Activity/Substance	Percentage of all cancer deaths
Smoking	30%
Diet	30%
Excessive growth early in life from overfeeding and low level of activity	5%
Genetics	5%
Occupational exposure	5%
Viruses and other infectious agents	5%
Reproduction related factors	4%
Alcohol	3%
Sedentary lifestyle	3%
Pollutants	2%
Radiation from the sun, electric power lines, household appliances, cellular phones, and radon gas	2%
Second-hand smoke	2%
Miscellaneous	2%
Food additives, mainly salt	1%
Medical products and procedures	1%

Additional Resources
for Cancer Information

American Cancer Society
The American Cancer society offers free booklets, education, and many services to patients and their families.
    1599 Clifton Rd., NE
    Atlanta, GA 30329
    1-800-227-2345
    www.cancer.org

One of the very best, easiest to understand books available on cancer diagnosis, treatment, and recovery is produced by the American Cancer Society. *Informed Decisions* is available through your local bookstore.

National Cancer Institute. A trained staff member can provide confidential answers to questions and mail you NCI publications. The National Cancer Institute also makes available the Physician Data Query (PDQ), a computerized database for doctors providing quick access to the most recent cancer treatment information.
    1-800-422-6237
    www.cancer.gov

American Institute for Cancer Research
Their nutrition hotline will answer your diet and cancer questions. A list of free brochures on healthy eating is also available.
    1759 R St., NW
    Washington, DC 20009
    202-328-7744

University of Pennsylvania Cancer Center
One of the most extensive, detailed, reliable source of information available on cancer. Varied topics include everything from personal experiences of cancer patients to discussion of new treatments to financial assistance programs.
    www.oncolink.upenn.edu

National Institute on Aging Information Center
Their information center can send free printed material about prostate problems, hospital stays, sexuality, and urinary incontinence.
    PO Box 8057
    Gaithersburg, MD 20898
    1-800-222-2225

National Stop Smoking Programs

American Institute for Preventive Medicine   800-345-2476
SMOKELESS

Smokstoppers   800-697-7221
   Web Site www.smokestoppers.com

Smokenders   800-828-4357

American Cancer Society   800-227-2345
FRESHSTART

American Lung Association   800-586-4872
FREEDOM FROM SMOKING
   Web Site www.lungusa.org

Nicotine Anonymous   415-750-0328
   Web Site www.nicotine-anonymous.org

www.quitsmokingsupport.com

PART
IV

THE
SECRETS
OF THE
PYRAMID

26

Forget the
Basic Four

You can decrease your fat intake, exercise, and still be in poor health because of the lack of *quality* in the food you're eating. You've heard about the basic four food groups for years, and that's still good information. But that system has been replaced with the food pyramid.

How much of each group in the pyramid you eat depends on the total number of calories you want to consume each day. A petite woman who eats only 1,500 calories a day to maintain her weight will eat less than a big macho guy who might be consuming 3,000 calories a day. Fortunately, you can go on line now to www.mypyramid.gov and get very specific guidelines. Just fill in your age, your gender, and your typical physical activity level and you'll get a pyramid designed just for you.

Figure 26.1

THE FOOD PYRAMID

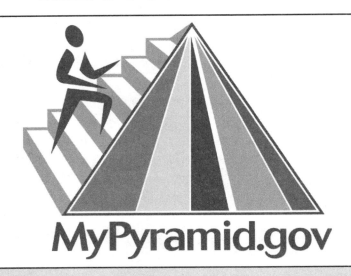

Find your balance between food and physical activity

- Be sure to stay within your daily calorie needs.
- Be physically active for at least 30 minutes most days of the week.
- About 60 minutes a day of physical activity may be needed to prevent weight gain.
- For sustaining weight loss, at least 60 to 90 minutes a day of physical activity may be required.
- Children and teenagers should be physically active for 60 minutes every day, or most days.

Know the limits on fats, sugars, and salt (sodium)

- Make most of your fat sources from fish, nuts, and vegetable oils.
- Limit solid fats like butter, stick margarine, shortening, and lard, as well as foods that contain these.
- Check the Nutrition Facts label to keep saturated fats, trans fats, and sodium low.
- Choose food and beverages low in added sugars. Added sugars contribute calories with few, if any, nutrients.

GRAINS Make half your grains whole

Eat at least 3 oz. of whole-grain cereals, breads, crackers, rice, or pasta every day 1 oz. is about 1 slice of bread, about 1 cup of breakfast cereal, or 1/2 cup of cooked rice, cereal, or pasta	**Eat 6 oz. every day**

VEGETABLES Vary your veggies

Eat more dark-green veggies like broccoli, spinach, and other dark leafy greens Eat more orange vegetables like carrots and sweetpotatoes Eat more dry beans and peas like pinto beans, kidney beans, and lentils	**Eat 2 1/2 cups every day**

FRUITS Focus on fruits

Eat a variety of fruit Choose fresh, frozen, canned, or dried fruit Go easy on fruit juices	**Eat 2 cups every day**

MILK Get your calcium-rich foods

Go low-fat or fat-free when you choose milk, yogurt, and other milk products If you don't or can't consume milk, choose lactose-free products or other calcium sources such as fortified foods and beverages	**Get 3 cups every day for kids aged 2 to 8, it's 2**

MEAT & BEANS Go lean with protein

Choose low-fat or lean meats and poultry Bake it, broil it, or grill it Vary your protein routine – choose more fish, beans, peas, nuts and seeds	**Eat 5 1/2 oz. every day**

For a 2,000-calorie intake, you need the amounts shown here for each food group. To find the amounts that are right for you, go to www.MyPyramid.gov

The Grain Group

Whether you're trying to improve your eating habits, to lose weight, or to just feel better, most of the food you consume every day should be from carbohydrates. Yes, carbohydrates! Breads, cereals, pastas, rice, and related foods all belong to this group. Fortunately, fat is really not a problem here. The only high-fat exceptions in breads are croissants, biscuits, and many commercially-made muffins.

Remember that even though fettuccine Alfredo, garlic bread, and fried rice all belong to this group, they're still high in fat. In each case it's not the fettuccine, bread, or rice that's the problem, but the fat that's been added.

Cereal is another carbohydrate food that's naturally low in fat. The only major exception is traditional granola. It's ironic that the one cereal that many people believe has a real health-food reputation is one of the few exceptions to an otherwise low-fat category. Fortunately, some manufacturers now offer lower-fat varieties of granola. As always, read the label for fat grams in a cereal you're considering.

Incidentally, to increase your fiber, look for breads and cereals that are made from *whole* wheat. Look for the words *whole wheat* to indicate that you're getting the complete food as God designed it. Some bread manufacturers would have you believe you're eating whole wheat even though they know better. *Wheat bread* is not much more than white bread with caramel coloring added. A bread labeled *wheat* only tells you the name of the plant that the bread comes from. *Wheat bread* only tells you there's no corn, barley, rice, or any other grain in the product. Other names that are misleading include *seven-grain, multi-grain, cracked wheat, stoneground,* and

> **M**ost of the food you consume every day should be from carbohydrates.

unbleached. All these names are simply trying to hide the fact that you've still got white bread. Don't be fooled, what you want is *whole* wheat, not just *wheat* bread. Whole wheat contains the fiber from the bran and the nutrition of the wheat germ. Wheat bread and white bread do not. While white bread—and for that matter *any* bread in the grocery store—is not bad for you, white bread is still man's idea. *Whole wheat* is God's idea.

> "**W**heat bread" is not much more than white bread with caramel coloring added.

Even though whole wheat is the best you can buy, there's another bread that's even better. See John 6:35–51.

Vegetables and Fruits

In this group try to emphasize those that are dark green or orange in color. Broccoli, carrots, and sweet potatoes are great choices to provide the antioxidant beta-carotene and other good nutrition.

Choose your favorite fruits, but make sure at least one is a citrus or some other fruit that provides vitamin C. Oranges and other citrus fruits, cantaloupes, and strawberries are good sources for your daily requirement of vitamin C.

Don't worry about the fat content in fruits and vegetables. The avocado is about the only item in this group that has fat. And even though olive oil is high in fat, a serving of olives themselves is not. It takes a whole lot of olives to make a tablespoon of olive oil. Even so, both avocados and olives contain the good unsaturated fats.

Of course, even though the potato is a great vegetable full of nutrition, when you turn it into french fries, the fat price tag goes up. The same goes for onion rings and for any other vegetable that you fry. Beyond these commonsense precautions, you can eat to your heart's content from the fruit and vegetable groups.

Go easy on fruit juices. Have you ever made fresh-squeezed orange juice? You have to go through a lot of oranges to get a good size glass of juice. While it's true that you get a lot of vitamin C, you're also getting a lot of sugar. When you eat a whole orange, on the other hand, you get great nutrition, fiber, and you control your sugar intake too.

Milk Group

If you haven't noticed already, the milk in your grocery store has undergone some name changes. What was formerly called *skim* is now referred to as *fat free*. What was formerly *1 percent* is now *low fat*, and the new name for *2 percent* milk is *reduced fat*. *Whole milk* will keep its same name. As a result, all you should be drinking is *low fat* or *fat free*.

If you're on whole milk now, begin to use reduced fat (2%). Eventually, though, you'll need to end up at low fat (1%) or fat free. I know, I know. I was raised on whole milk too. The first time I tasted fat free I thought it had spoiled! It took me a while to get used to it, but now that's all I drink. And it tastes *good* to me. I don't tolerate it anymore; I *like* it. It may take you a while too. That's okay. You have time. You don't have to get there by tomorrow.

> A gallon of whole milk contains a whopping 32 restaurant pats of butter!

When you drink one eight-ounce cup of whole milk, you're also swallowing two restaurant pats of butter. In the old days the cream used to separate and rise to the top. Now the milk is homogenized and you don't see the cream anymore. But it's all still in there.

A gallon of whole milk contains a whopping 32 restaurant pats of butter! And butter is animal fat. By this time you know how we feel about animal fat. You'll also shortly learn what God's Word has to say about animal fat too.

One eight-ounce cup of reduced fat (2%) milk contains one pat of butter. That's better than whole milk, but it's still not good enough. You've still got 16 pats of butter in each gallon of reduced fat (2%) milk.

Unfortunately, many people who drink reduced fat (2%) milk as part of their heart healthy diet program think they've arrived when in fact they're only on the way.

Switch to low fat (1%) milk and *now* you're making a real difference. Low fat (1%) milk only contains a half pat of butter per cup. That's a substantial step in the right direction. Fat free milk takes it a step further.

If it takes you some time to get to fat free milk, that's fine. But remember that fat free is perfection, and your goal is *moderation*. The half a pat of butter per cup in low fat (1%) milk is enough to still give it some flavor. For those people who absolutely refuse to drink fat free milk, that's good enough. At low fat (1%) milk you've dramatically cut your fat content from whole milk and still have a little flavor. If you already drink fat free milk, that's even better.

Cheese is notoriously high in fat. Fortunately, there are many lower-fat cheese products available now. Again, read the label for fat grams. Using sharp cheese whenever you can will allow you to use a smaller quantity of cheese and still have the flavor. More flavor, less cheese needed.

By the way, if you have trouble digesting dairy products try lactose-free products or other calcium sources like soy milk.

Meat & Beans

Today it's more appropriate to talk about the protein group rather than the meat group. If you eat meat, make sure it's very lean. Also, watch the amount of meat you eat at any one time. A 12-ounce steak may taste good, but that's enough protein for your body for two entire days—and it often comes with a very high-fat price tag. Instead of making your meal revolve around meat, put meat *in* the recipe—as part of the dish. Chinese and Italian cooks have been doing this for years, and with very positive health benefits. You don't have to stop eating meat, just cut down on how *much* you eat and how *often* you eat it.

> Instead of making your meal revolve around meat, put meat *in* the recipe—as part of the dish.

Based upon how much fat they contain, beef, veal, and lamb come in three grades: prime, choice, and select. *Prime* is the fattest and thus the juiciest and most tender. But that's not juice—it's grease!

Choice is lower in fat content, and *Select* is the lowest of all. Go with the select grade whenever you can. To make the meat more tender, don't overcook it. You might also marinate it overnight using a recipe that includes something like lemon juice or vinegar as an ingredient. The acid helps break down the protein in the meat and makes it more tender. The *round* cut of the animal is one of the leanest. Some examples of lower-fat cuts of beef include top round, eye of round, round steak, rump roast, sirloin tip, short loin, and ground sirloin.

A suggested three-ounce broiled portion of 80 percent lean ground beef has 15 grams of fat; 85 percent lean has 12 grams. Leaner hamburger is more expensive per pound because you're getting more meat and less fat. When you cook leaner hamburger you'll get much less grease.

Surprisingly, a three-ounce serving of ground turkey can have the same amount of fat as leaner hamburger. Why is ground turkey so high? Because meat processors include the dark meat as well as the skin. Be sure to look for the fat gram listing on the label of the ground turkey you buy.

Hot dogs and luncheon meats are not only very high in

salt, but they're often loaded with fat. Read the label!

Don't forget chicken. A three-ounce baked chicken leg with the skin has 15 grams of fat; without the skin it only has eight. The same size serving of a baked chicken thigh with the skin has 10 grams of fat. Remove the skin, and the fat grams go down to six. If you take the skin off chicken you get rid of a lot of the fat and significantly cut the calories too.

A three-ounce skinless baked chicken breast only has about three grams of fat. By removing the skin you can afford to eat more chicken for the same number of calories. Wouldn't you rather have more food than less?

Almost all supermarkets now post the nutritional value and fat content of all beef, poultry, and fish items. If there's not an actual nutrition label on the meat you're buying, ask the butcher for the specific information you want.

Fish, dry beans, and peas are also part of the protein group. Not only are beans and peas good for protein, they're also high in carbohydrates, fiber, vitamins, minerals, and low in fat. They're a lot less expensive than meat too. That is, unless your name is Esau.

You may remember that in Genesis 25:34 Esau gave his birthright over to Jacob in exchange for lentil stew and bread. That was the

> The most expensive meal in history.
> *Genesis 25:34*

most expensive meal in history. But at least it was nutritious! Today you shouldn't have to pay nearly as much. Beans, peas, and lentils usually go for around 89¢ a bag. Try to have a meal with beans instead of meat at least twice a week.

Oils & Fats

The smallest section of the food pyramid is occupied by oils and fats. Solid fats like butter and liquid vegetable oils are, of course, fat. As you know, saturated fats (cream, butter, lard), the tropical oils (palm, palm kernel, coconut), and trans fats (found in foods that have been partially hydrogenated) are the real problem. But getting the fat you eat from the unsaturated vegetable oils (like olive, peanut, or canola) or the omega-3 fish oils may be a good decision. Surprisingly, a recent study showed that a nutritious diet that included some extra olive oil helped reduce heart disease risk even better than a very low total-fat diet did. Those with diabetes or high triglycerides may also benefit from eating a little more of these good fats too; just remember to keep your calories under control.

Of the fat you do eat, get it from vegetable oils, nuts, and fish. The current guidelines recommend that anywhere from 20-35% of the total calories you eat can come from fat. For a 2,000 calorie daily intake that comes to anywhere from 44 to 78 grams of fat. As I said back in Chapter 4, I think 50 grams a day is a good target for most people.

27

The Dietary Guidelines For Americans

You sure hear a lot of different opinions when it comes to health. People are confused. They don't know what to believe any more. Fortunately, every five years the US government publishes guidelines to promote good nutrition and prevent diseases. You *can* trust the following guidelines to put you and your family on the road to great health.

Eat *Quality* Foods

Choose a diet with plenty of whole grain products, vegetables, and fruits. And to get the energy, protein, vitamins, minerals, and fiber you need for good health, eat a lot of different foods. Since no one food has all the nutrients your body requires, you need to consume a great variety.

Keep in mind that there is no perfect food. Manna was the

> Moderation is the foundation upon which nutrition and good health are built.

only food that had everything that a human needed for good health (Exodus 16; Numbers 11), but you can't get it anymore! There's really no such thing as a junk food either. True, a lot of foods in the supermarket have very little nutritional value, but none of them — as some people would imply — are poison. What *will* impact your health is how often and how much of a particular food you eat. *Frequency* and *quantity* are the key words to remember.

Now you certainly don't have to become a vegetarian to be healthy. But you probably do need to eat less meat than the average American currently consumes. Keep in mind, though, that children, teenage girls, and women in their childbearing years need to emphasize iron-rich foods like lean meats and iron-fortified foods like cereal and breads.

Teenage girls and women also need to be sure they get enough calcium to build and maintain strong bones to help ward off osteoporosis. Low-fat and fat free dairy products are the most efficient source of calcium. Folic acid, one of the B vitamins, is also very important for women in their childbearing years. Fortunately, it's now added to many foods.

People over fifty should be sure they get enough vitamin B12 either in fortified foods or supplements. Look for 100% of the Daily Value for B12 on your supplement label. Vitamin D is also often low in older people, those with dark skin, and those that don't get enough sunlight. 400-800 IU of vitamin D is a good daily goal.

Fiber is important for everyone. You need both the soluble fiber found in oats, dried beans, fruits, and vegetables and the insoluble fiber found in whole grain products for good health. Try to make at least half the breads and cereals you eat *whole* grain. You want *whole* wheat bread, not wheat bread.

Some people say that the quality of nutrition in our foods isn't what it was 100 years ago. They suggest that an orange, for example, doesn't have the good nutrition it used to have. Even if that was true, at least you can *get* an orange in the dead of winter in Minnesota today.

In the "good old days," people got scurvy and other life-threatening problems because they didn't even have access to foods. Today you can get a wide variety of food whenever you want it, 12 months a year. The real problem is actually getting people to eat the good quality food that's available.

Watch Your Fat Intake

As we've already said many times, reducing your risk of heart attack and cancer is your highest health priority. Make sure that most of the fat you eat comes from plant, not animal, sources. Nuts and vegetable oils are good choices. Though technically an "animal," the fat and oil in fish is healthy too. The official recommendation is that no more than ten percent of the calories you consume be from the artery-clogging saturated fat. That means that if you eat about 2000 calories a day, your saturated fat intake shouldn't go above about 20 grams. Reducing your intake of foods high in cholesterol like egg yolks and organ meats (like liver) also helps. Trans fats can also be a problem. They're often found in commercially baked goods like cookies and crackers and also stick margarine and fast food french fries. Be watching the updated food label for specific listings of trans fats. The less the better.

A 2,000 calorie daily intake will mean that your saturated fat intake shouldn't exceed 20 grams.

Remember too, that a reduced fat diet can also help you maintain a healthy weight.

Go Easy On The Sugar Bowl

A diet high in sugar can have too many calories and too few nutrients for most people. Is sugar poison? No. Is it good for you? No. But it sure helps make life a little more enjoyable.

The evidence against fat is far greater than the case against sugar. So what's the recommended intake of sugar? There is none. To give a recommendation for sugar would imply that you have a physiological need for sugar. But your body can live just fine without it. You *do* need some fat, sodium, and fiber every day for your health, but you have no need for sugar.

America's consumption of soft drinks is up 85% in the last twenty years. Each man, woman, and child now consumes an average of more than 50 gallons a year—America's number one source of sugar.

You may have a *psychological* need for sugar, but that's just a perceived need—not a requirement of your body. Nevertheless, you can still use the food label to figure how much sugar you're getting in a product.

One teaspoon of sugar in a food is equal to a listing of 4 grams of sugar on the nutrition label. If you find that one serving of a product has 40 grams listed as sugar, that's the same thing as 10 teaspoons! Even though there's no official recommendation, common sense should tell you that that particular product is very high in sugar.

Incidentally, brown sugar is no better for you than white sugar. They make brown sugar from white simply by mixing it with a little syrup or molasses. Don't be fooled into thinking brown sugar is better for you—it's just sugar. And even though we've said that sugar is not the real enemy, it still doesn't do you any good. The average American is taking in over 42 pounds of the white substance every year. You'll be better off decreasing your intake.

Eat Less Salt and More Potassium

Remember that the salt shaker can be your friend! To help reduce your risk of high blood pressure, *put it back on the table!* At the same time get educated about the real source of salt—the supermarket. People with high blood pressure, those fifty and above, and blacks should try to limit their sodium intake to no more than 1500 mg per day. That won't be easy! Getting more potassium sources like fruits and vegetables and dairy products can help too. The recommended target for potassium is 4700 mg a day. And don't forget that losing excess body fat may be all you really need to do to get your blood pressure back to normal again.

Get Moving!

To reduce your chances of obesity, high blood pressure, heart disease, stroke, certain cancers, and the most common form of diabetes, you need physical activity in your lifestyle. That's why there's a picture of a person exercising on the side of the food pyramid. You were designed by your Creator to *move*.

The current guidelines are to get anywhere from 30-90 minutes of exercise on most days. Most people aren't anywhere close to that. In general, the more vigorous and the longer you go, the better. A good fitness program consists of three components: cardiovascular, stretching for flexibility, and resistive exercise for muscular strength.

Nutrition by itself is not the answer. Physical activity by itself is not the answer either. For optimal health you need both. Make sure the activity you choose for exercise is both convenient and *fun!*

Easy On The Alcohol

Some evidence suggests that moderate alcohol consumption of no more than two drinks a day for a man or one drink a day for a woman may decrease your heart disease risk. Other studies show that when you drink alcohol you increase your risk of breast and other cancers and for cirrhosis of the liver.

Women in their childbearing years who may become pregnant, pregnant and breastfeeding women, and those taking certain medications that can interact with alcohol should all avoid it.

Alcohol is a loaded gun. Lives and families can be destroyed when it gets into the wrong hands. You can take many other positive, *no-risk* steps to prevent heart disease. Consuming alcohol for "health reasons" is most likely not the best decision. If you do drink, keep it moderate. If you don't, don't start.

Keep It Clean

Obviously food that makes you sick isn't going to do you any good. Millions of people suffer from food poisoning every year in this country. Not only is it inconvenient and uncomfortable, but it can be very dangerous for those whose immune systems aren't healthy. This is especially true for young children, pregnant women, and older adults. Make sure your food is always cooked thoroughly, defrost it in the refrigerator, and avoid unpasteurized milk, uncooked eggs, and raw seafood.

Figure 27.1

THE RULES TO THE GAME

There's a game going on in your supermarket. The game is between you the consumer and the food manufacturers. The food manufacturers' goal is to see what they can get you to buy. Your goal is to maintain and improve your and your family's health. The average consumer is bombarded with advertising and marketing and hasn't got a chance to win the game without knowing what the rules are. Now *you* have a chance.

SUGGESTED DAILY DIETARY INTAKE FOR ADULTS

Total Fat . . . . **50 grams or less**

Saturated Fat . . . . . **20 grams or less**
(This 20 grams *is part* of your total 50 grams allowance, not in addition to it.)

Sodium . . . . **1,500-2,300 mg or less**

Potassium . . . . **4,700 mg**

Fiber . . . . **30 grams**

Sugar . . . . **1 teaspoon = 4 grams***

Cholesterol . . . . **300 mg or less**

*A conversion factor only; there is no suggested dietary intake for sugar.

Please remember, the *total* number of calories you eat *is* important! However, a goal for calories is not listed here since simply counting calories can still potentially result in a low calorie, high-fat, and high-sugar diet. If, on the other hand—since there are more calories in a gram of fat than anything else—you count grams of fat and don't go wild with sugar, calories automatically will come down. Counting fat grams rather than calories is a much more efficient way to control your calorie intake.

Figure 27.2

THE FOOD LABEL AT A GLANCE

Serving sizes are now more consistent across product lines and are stated in both household and metric measures. But be careful. Many products still list a serving size that is much smaller than what you probably eat. That makes the rest of the numbers look better than what you're really getting.

The list of nutrients covers those most important to the health of today's consumers, most of whom need to be concerned about getting *too much* of certain items (fat, for example) rather than too few vitamins or minerals, as in the past.

Nutrition Facts

Serving Size 3 cookies (34g/1.2 oz)
Servings per container About 5

Amount per serving
Calories 180   Calories from Fat 90

	%Daily Value*
Total Fat 10 g	**15%**
Saturated Fat 3.5g	**18%**
Trans Fat 3g	
Polyunsaturated Fat 1g	
Monounsaturated Fat 2.5g	
Cholesterol 10mg	**3%**
Sodium 80mg	**3%**
Total Carbohydrate 21g	**7%**
Dietary Fiber 1g	**4%**
Sugars 11g	
Protein 2g	

Vitamin A 0%	•	Vitamin C 0%	
Calcium 0%	•	Iron 4%	
Thiamin 6%	•	Riboflavin 4%	
Niacin 4%			

* Percent Daily Values are based on a 2,000 calorie diet. Your daily values may be higher or lower depending on your caloric needs:

	Calories	2,000	2,500
Total Fat	Less than:	65g	80g
Sat Fat	Less than	20g	25g
Cholesterol	Less than	2,400mg	2,400mg
Total Carbohydrate		300g	375g
Dietary Fiber		25g	30g

Ingredients: Unbleached enriched wheat flour [flour, niacin, reduced iron, thiamin, mononitrate (vitamin B1)], sweet chocolate (sugar, chocolate liquor, cocoa butter, soy lecithin added as an emulaifier, vanilla extract), sugar, partially hydrogenated vegetable shortening (soybean, cottonseed and/or canola oils), nonfat milk, whole eggs, cornstarch, egg whites, salt vanilla extract, baking soda and soy lecithin.

The main number to be watching for is that of the fat grams. Also, the fewer the saturated fat grams, the better.

% Daily Value shows how a food fits into the overall daily diet. For example, one serving of this food (3 cookies) will provide you with **4%** of the fiber you need for the day.

Some Daily Values are maximums, as with fat (65 grams or less); others are minimums, as with carbohydrate (300 grams or more). But don't worry about counting carbohydrates.

The daily values for a 2,000-and a 2,500-calorie diet are listed. In my opinion the recommended fat intake is still too liberal. Just use the Rules To The Game guidelines on page 195.

ACTION STEPS
FOR IMPROVED NUTRITION

1. **Eat more carbohydrates than anything else!** Breads, cereals, pasta, and rice are the foundation upon which a healthy food intake is based. Remember, most of the world lives on carbohydrates, and they're not fat. Obesity's not near the problem in China as it is here, and they eat *a lot* of rice!

2. **Of the carbohydrates you do eat, make them whole grain whenever possible.** Remember, you want *whole wheat* bread, not just *wheat* bread. Brown rice is whole grain; white rice is not.

3. **For good nutrition, eat the recommended number of servings from each food group of the food pyramid and follow the Dietary Guidelines for Americans.**

4. **Memorize "The Rules To The Game."** Use them as the standard when you evaluate a particular food from its food label. Remember, any food can fit into a healthy diet. It's how often you eat it and how much of it you consume that matters.

V

WHAT THE BIBLE SAYS ABOUT WHAT YOU EAT

28

Just for Israel?

Some would say that the Old Testament dietary laws were only for the nation of Israel, that the Jews were God's chosen people, and that God created specific regulations and laws so that they would be a holy people, different from the rest of the sinful world.

But that was for the Jews. It wasn't for the rest of the world; and it's certainly not for Christians today. Some would say "We don't have to follow all these rules; after all, we are free through Jesus Christ." I agree. We don't *have to* follow the Old Testament dietary laws—we are indeed free through Jesus Christ. Nevertheless, we might still *want to* follow them.

Everybody on the Boat!

How many animals of each kind did Noah take on the ark? Two, right? Well, I thought it was two also, until I saw Genesis 7:2:

> Take with you *seven* of every kind of *clean animal*, a male and its mate, and *two* of every kind of *unclean animal*.

Did you know that was in there? I never did. We've all seen the little Sunday school story pictures, with two animals, side by side. Well, those must have been the unclean ones going in; the clean animals must have already been on the boat!

Why would God tell Noah to take seven of every kind of clean animal, but to bring only two of every kind of unclean animal? Could it be that God recognized the need for Noah and his family to have animals for both food and sacrifice after the flood?

How many of each animal did Noah take on the ark?

Keep in mind that all plant life was also destroyed in the flood and that Noah and his family had to have something to eat. Furthermore, it would not have been appropriate for Noah to offer up an unclean animal as a thanksgiving offering to God for His provision.

So God provided for seven of each kind of clean animal to survive, both for Noah's needs and for the continuation of the species. But God only provided for two of each unclean animal, simply to make sure they survived the flood.

Here are some questions to consider: Where is the nation of Israel at the time of the flood? Nowhere! It doesn't exist yet. Has Abraham been born? Not yet. Has Moses received the Ten Commandments? No—he hasn't been born yet either. And yet, clean and unclean animals were already identified.

It appears that Noah knew which were which. The Lord told him to choose seven of the *clean* and two of the *unclean*. God seems to have identified certain foods that man would do best to avoid from very early on. *And it appears that God identified those foods long before we see their specific application to the nation of Israel.*

The wisdom of the clean and unclean foods may, therefore, not be limited only to the nation of Israel. This wisdom may, in fact, have application for all of God's people, regardless of when they lived, even those of us living today.

Whose Fat Is It, Anyway?

As a nutritionist, if there is one bottom-line health message I deliver as I speak, it is to "eat less fat." Especially to "eat less saturated animal fat." You know that by now. You also know that fat from vegetables and plant sources—while it's still loaded with calories—can be a part of healthful eating. Saturated animal fat contributes dramatically to the number one killer today—heart disease. Animal fat just doesn't seem to agree with us humans. Consider what God's Word has to say about this issue:

- "This is a lasting ordinance for the generations to come, wherever you live: You must not eat any fat or any blood." (Leviticus 3:17). If you read the Scripture in the context of the chapter, it's clear God is prohibiting animal fat specifically.

- "The LORD said to Moses, 'Say to the Israelites: "Do not eat any of the fat of cattle, sheep or goats." '" (Leviticus 7:22–23). Scripture is clear that animal fat is not to be used for human consumption.

- "The priest shall burn them on the altar as food, an offering made by fire, a pleasing aroma. *All the fat is the LORD's*" (Leviticus 3:16).

- "The priest is to sprinkle the blood against the altar of the LORD at the entrance of the Tent of Meeting and *burn the fat as an aroma pleasing to the LORD*" (Leviticus 17:6).

- "Now Abel kept flocks, and Cain worked the soil. In the course of time Cain brought some of the fruits of the soil as an offering to the LORD. *But Abel brought fat portions from some of the firstborn of his flock. The LORD looked with favor on Abel and his offering*, but on Cain and his offering he did not look with favor. So Cain was very angry, and his face was downcast. Then the LORD said to Cain, 'Why are you angry? Why is your face downcast? *If you do what is right*, will you not be accepted?' " (Genesis 4:2).

- "Since you eat meat with the blood still in it . . . should you then possess the land?" (Ezekiel 33:25). This is one of the reasons Israel was taken into captivity and lost the promised land.

- "Eli's sons were wicked men; they had no regard for the Lord. Now it was the practice of the priests with the people that whenever anyone offered a sacrifice and while the meat was being boiled, the servant of the priest would come with the three-pronged fork in his hand. He would plunge it into the pan or kettle or cauldron or pot, and the priest would take for himself whatever the fork brought up. This is how they treated all the Israelites that came to Shiloh. *But even before the fat was burned,* the servant of the priests would come and say to the man who was sacrificing, 'Give the priest some meat to roast; he won't accept boiled meat from you, but only raw.' If the man said to him, 'Listen, let the fat be burned up first, and then take whatever you want,' the servant would then answer, 'No, hand it over now; If you don't, I will take it by force.' *This sin of the young men was very great in the Lord's sight,* for they were treating the Lord's offering with contempt" (1 Samuel 2:12–17). In what way were they sinning? They were eating the meat with the fat still on it.

- "[The Israelites] pounced on the plunder and, taking sheep, cattle and calves, they butchered them on the ground and ate them, together with the blood. Then someone said to Saul, "Look, the men are sinning against the LORD by eating meat that has blood in it"" (1 Samuel 14:32–33a).

It goes without saying that we would never eat blood today. The idea is disgusting. It almost suggests some type of satanic involvement. If it were discovered that someone at your church was drinking blood, a special meeting of the pastor and church leadership would most likely be called. This kind of activity would be addressed quickly and decisively. We seem to know in our very beings that eating blood is unacceptable.

As we've seen in Leviticus 3:17, in God's sight, *eating animal fat* is just as unacceptable. And that prohibition is for all the generations. Consuming blood would cause real indignation in your church, and yet eating animal fat is practiced by many church members today without any thought whatsoever. It may be that animal fat was never designed for human consumption. We may be better off just not eating it.

> It may be that animal fat was never designed for human consumption.

29

For Us Today?

Are the dietary laws *really* for people today? A part of Scripture that is very often misunderstood is the meaning of Peter's vision in Acts 10:1–35. Many today will cite this as proof positive that the Lord said all foods are now clean and okay to eat. Let's see what it really says.

- **Peter's Vision, Acts 10:1–35**

  At Caesarea there was a man named Cornelius, a centurion in what was known as the Italian regiment. He and all his family were devout and God-fearing; he gave generously to those in need and prayed to God regularly. One day at about three in the afternoon he had a vision. He distinctly saw an angel of God, who came to him and said, "Cornelius!"

  Cornelius stared at him in fear. "What is it, Lord?" he asked.

  The angel answered, "Your prayers and gifts to the poor have come up as a memorial offering before God. Now send men to Joppa to bring back a man named

Simon who is called Peter. He is staying with Simon the tanner, whose house is by the sea."

When the angel who spoke to him had gone, Cornelius called two of his servants and a devout soldier who was one of his attendants. He told them everything that had happened and sent them to Joppa.

About noon the following day as they were on their journey and approaching the city, Peter went up on the roof to pray. He became hungry and wanted something to eat, and while the meal was being prepared, he fell into a trance. He saw heaven opened and something like a large sheet being let down to earth by its four corners. It contained all kinds of four-footed animals, as well as reptiles of the earth and birds of the air. Then a voice told him, "Get up, Peter. Kill and eat."

"Surely not, Lord!" Peter replied. "I have never eaten anything impure or unclean."

The voice spoke to him a second time, "Do not call anything impure that God has made clean."

This happened three times, and immediately the sheet was taken back to heaven.

While Peter was wondering about the meaning of the vision, the men sent by Cornelius found out where Simon's house was and stopped at the gate. They called out, asking if Simon who was known as Peter was staying there.

While Peter was still thinking about the vision, the Spirit said to him, "Simon, three men are looking for you. So get up and go downstairs. Do not hesitate to go with them, for I have sent them."

Peter went down and said to the men, "I'm the one you're looking for. Why have you come?"

The men replied, "We have come from Cornelius the centurion. He is a righteous and God-fearing man, who is respected by all the Jewish people. A holy angel told him to have you come to his house so that he could hear what you have to say." Then Peter invited the men into the house to be his guests.

The next day Peter started out with them, and some of the brothers from Joppa went along. The following day he arrived in Caesarea. Cornelius was expecting them and had called together his relatives and close friends. As Peter entered the house, Cornelius met him and fell at his feet in reverence. But Peter made him get up. "Stand up," he said, "I am only a man myself."

Talking with him, Peter went inside and found a large gathering of people. He said to them: ***"You are well aware that it is against our law for a Jew to associate with a Gentile or visit him. But God has shown me that I should not call any man impure or unclean.*** So when I was sent for, I came without raising any objection. May I ask why you sent for me?"

Cornelius answered: "Four days ago I was in my house praying at this hour, at three in the afternoon. Suddenly a man in shining clothes stood before me and said, 'Cornelius, God has heard your prayer and remembered your gifts to the poor. Send to Joppa for Simon who is called Peter. He is a guest in the home of Simon the tanner, who lives by the sea.' So I sent for you immediately, and it was good of you to come. Now we are all here in the presence of God to listen to everything the Lord has commanded you to tell us."

Then Peter began to speak: "I now realize how true it is that God does not show favoritism but accepts men from every nation who fear him and do what is right."

Peter's vision has *nothing* to do with clean and unclean foods! It was clear to Peter that the Lord was now welcoming the so-called unclean Gentiles into the family of God. That's what the lesson is all about. No longer was there to be a spiritual separation. Jews and Gentiles were both now to be spiritual brothers through Jesus Christ.

When some of Peter's fellow Jewish believers became upset when they heard that Peter had entered the home of unclean Gentiles, he reconfirmed the message. They were soon in agreement with Peter:

When they heard this, they had no further objections and praised God, saying, "So then, God has granted even the Gentiles repentance unto life" (Acts 11:18).

• **Did Jesus Really Say That All Foods Are Clean?** Look at **Mark 7:5–23:**

So the Pharisees and teachers of the law asked Jesus, "Why don't your disciples live according to the tradition of the elders instead of eating their food with 'unclean' hands?"

He replied, "Isaiah was right when he prophesied about you hypocrites; as it is written:

'These people honor me with their lips,

but their hearts are far from me.

They worship me in vain;

their teachings are but rules taught by men.'

You have let go of the commands of God and are holding on to the traditions of men."

And he said to them: "You have a fine way of setting aside the commands of God in order to observe your own traditions! For Moses said, 'Honor your father and your mother,' and, 'Anyone who curses his father or mother must be put to death.' But you say that if a man says to his father or mother: 'Whatever help you might otherwise have received from me is 'Corban' (that is, a gift devoted to God), then you no longer let him do anything for his father or mother. Thus you nullify the word of God by your tradition that you have handed down. And you do many things like that."

Again Jesus called the crowd to him and said, "Listen to me, everyone, and understand this. Nothing outside a man can make him 'unclean' by going into him. Rather, it is what comes out of a man that makes him 'unclean.'"

After he had left the crowd and entered the house, his disciples asked him about this parable. "Are you so dull?" he asked. "Don't you see that nothing that enters a man from the outside can make him 'unclean'? For it doesn't go into his heart but into his stomach, and then out of his body." (In saying this, Jesus declared all foods "clean.")

He went on: "What comes out of a man is what makes him 'unclean.' For from within, out of men's hearts, come evil thoughts, sexual immorality, theft, murder, adultery, greed, malice, deceit, lewdness, envy, slander, arrogance and folly. All these evils come from inside and make a man "unclean.'"

Jesus was identifying the hypocrisy of the Jews, who were so concerned about Jesus' disciples following Jewish tradition that they missed the point and intention of God's Word.

The tradition of the time allowed a Jew to designate all of his possessions for the work of God (Corban). That, in itself, was not a bad idea. But in doing so the Jewish tradition also said he was now free of any obligation to take care of his parents in their old age.

Jesus said that *that* was a problem of the heart. God's command to honor your father and mother was still superior to any Jewish tradition, regardless of its good intent. Some Jews were using the good tradition to avoid God's command.

Jesus' concern was of the internal sinful nature, and yet the Jews were worried about the outward traditional washing of hands in a ceremonial ritual. Jesus was saying that whether you wash your hands or don't wash your hands doesn't make you a clean or unclean person. What comes from inside your heart is what matters.

In some translations, the NIV included, there is a parenthetical statement at the end of verse 19: "(In saying this, Jesus declared all foods 'clean')." Is that *really* what Jesus said?

If you reread the chapter, you'll see that Jesus was identifying the hypocrisy of the Jews. He was *not* talking about whether formerly unclean foods would now be clean. The issue of food is not even addressed.

Interestingly, there is no parenthetical statement in the same story in Matthew 15:1–20, and the incident isn't even addressed in Luke or John. Even more important is the fact that the parenthetical statement is nowhere to be found at all in the original Greek (Mark 7:17–23):

17 Καὶ ὅτε εἰσῆλθεν εἰς οἶκον ἀπὸ τοῦ ὄχλου, ἐπηρώτων αὐτον
And   when   he entered   into   a house   from   the   crowd,   questioned   him

οἱ μαθηταὶ αὐτοῦ τὴν παραβολήν.
the   disciples   of him   the   parable.

18 καὶ λέγει αὐτοῖς οὕτως καὶ ὑμεῖς ἀσύνετοί ἐστε; οὐ νοεῖτε
And   he says   to them: Thus   also   you   undiscerning   are?   Do you not understand

ὅτι πᾶν τὸ ἔξωθεν εἰσπορευόμενον εἰς τὸν ἄνθρωπον οὐ δύναται
that everything from without   entering   into -----   a man   cannot

αὐτὸν κοινῶσαι,
him   to defile,

19 ὅτι οὐκ εἰσπορεύεται αὐτοῦ εἰς τὴν καρδίαν ἀλλ' εἰς
because   it enters not   of him   into   the   heart   but   into

τὴν κοιλίαν, καὶ εἰς τὸν ἀφεδρῶνα ἐκπορεύεται,
the   belly,   and   into   the   drain   goes out,

καθαρίζων πάντα τὰ βρώματα
purging   all   ---   foods?

20 ἔλεγεν δὲ ὅτι τὸ ἐκ τοῦ ἀνθρώπου ἐκπορευόμενον,
And he said (,) --- the thing out of --   a man   coming forth,

ἐκεῖνο κοινοῖ τὸν ἄνθρωπον.
that   defiles   ----,   a man.

21 ἔσωθεν γὰρ ἐκ τῆς καρδίας τῶν ἀνθρώπων οἱ διαλογισμοὶ οἱ
from within   for   out of the   heart   ---   of men   ---   thoughts   ---

κακοὶ ἐκπορεύονται, πορνεῖαι, κλοπαί, φόνοι,
evil   come forth,   fornications,   thefts,   murders,

22 μοιχεῖαι, πλεονεξίαι, πονηρίαι, δόλος, ἀσέλγεια,
adulteries, greediness, iniquities, deceit, lewdness,

ὀφθαλμὸς πονηρός, βλασφημία, ὑπερηφανία, ἀφροσύνη
eye wicked, blasphemy, arrogance, foolishness;

23 πάντα ταῦτα τὰ πονηρὰ ἔσωθεν ἐκπορεύεται καὶ
all these ---- evil things from within comes forth and

κοινοῖ τὸν ἄνθρωπον.
defile ----- a man.

It's clear from the original text that Jesus was not discussing clean and unclean foods at all. So where did the parenthetical statement— "In saying this, Jesus declared all foods clean"— come from? Somewhere along the way those who translated the Scripture from the original Greek may have inserted their commentary in the form of the parenthetical statement. That's why it's in parentheses—to indicate commentary.

So how could the translator of Mark make such a conclusion when it's clear upon reading the text that indeed Jesus was talking about unclean character coming from the heart, not from food? It may hinge on the word *purge* found in verse 19, "*purging* all foods."

Even today some would say that *purging* implies that the body cleansed the foods when eaten. To me, however, the word *purge* means "to remove, to get rid of." If information is purged from a computer, it's removed. The quality of the information is not improved or cleaned up.

It's interesting to note that the Greek word for *purge*, καθαρίζω (*katharidzo*), is also found in Hebrews 1:3: "The Son is the radiance of God's glory and the exact representation of his being, sustaining all things by his powerful word. After he had provided *purification* (καθαρισμον) for sins, he sat down at the right hand of the Majesty in heaven."

Here the word is translated "purification." But is that really what Jesus has done to our sins? Has He simply cleaned them up? We still have them, but they're now just clean? Hardly.

Scripture says we are a new creation (2 Corinthians 5:17). Our sins are now as far from us as the east is from the west (Psalm 103:12). The sins of our past are not cleansed; they are done away with. In the same manner, when our body purges our food it doesn't cleanse it, it gets rid of it. Our body doesn't clean foods; it just sends them through the system.

The parenthetical comment that Jesus declared all foods clean doesn't seem to fit with what the Bible really says.

• **Faith, Not Religion**

Another Scripture that often is confusing is found in **Colossians 2:16–23**:

Therefore do not let anyone judge you by what you eat or drink, or with regard to a religious festival, a New Moon celebration or a Sabbath day. These are a shadow of the things that were to come; the reality, however, is found in Christ. Do not let anyone who delights in false humility and the worship of angels disqualify you for the prize. Such a person goes into great detail about what he has seen, and his unspiritual mind puffs him up with idle notions. He has lost connection with the Head, from whom the whole body, supported and held together by its ligaments and sinews, grows as God causes it to grow.

Since you died with Christ to the basic principles of this world, why, as though you still belonged to it, do you submit to its rules: "Do not handle! Do not taste! Do not touch!"? These are all destined to perish with use, because they are based on human commands and teachings. Such regulations indeed have an appearance of wisdom, with their self-imposed worship, their false humility and their harsh treatment of the body, but they lack any value in restraining sensual indulgence.

When Paul wrote the letter to the Colossians there was a great deal of heresy arising in the young church. Certain groups were adding requirements and distorting the simple message of salvation through faith.

Yes, you needed faith in Jesus Christ, but you also still needed to be circumcised. Yes, you needed faith in Jesus Christ, but you also were required to observe special ceremonies or avoid certain foods. Their faith had become a religion; a list of things to do and not do. People were judged on whether or not they were following the rules.

Paul attacked that deception.

In *Eating By The Book* we're not talking about judgment, but rather opportunity. The opportunity to physically benefit from the wisdom of God's Word.

Paul continued the same thought in **1 Timothy 4:3–5**:

> They forbid people to marry and order them to abstain from certain foods, which God created to be received with thanksgiving by those who believe and who know the truth. For everything God created is good, and nothing is to be rejected if it is received with thanksgiving, because it is consecrated by the word of God and prayer.

Once again Paul addresses this issue, this time to Timothy. Paul felt obligated to identify and correct this deception of "salvation with conditions" before it had any further impact on the young Christian church.

This Scripture also brings up another interesting idea. Were unclean foods—those foods that were not to be consumed, as God revealed through Moses— created "to be received with thanksgiving"? Was the pig to be received with thanksgiving? I don't think so.

It's true that all things that God created are good, but that

> **S**o whether you eat or drink or whatever you do, do it all for the glory of God.
> *1 Corinthians 10:31*

doesn't necessarily mean that they were all created to be eaten. The pig and the vulture were both created for a good purpose, but not necessarily for human consumption. In my opinion, Paul is warning Timothy against the people who are telling others that formerly *clean* foods are now to be avoided.

Paul also says that the Word of God and prayer consecrate food. If he was indeed talking about the clean foods as revealed through God's Word, then that makes sense. But my dad prayed over the food he ate as far back as I can remember, both before and after meals. Did that change the very nature of the high-fat pork and other foods that he consumed? Did that change the quality and the content of the food that contributed to his early death at age 56? I can't see that it did.

- **You're Free to Eat Whatever You Want.**
  In **Romans 14:14** Paul wrote, "I am fully convinced that no food is unclean in itself." I agree. From a spiritual standpoint, no food is unclean. But that's all Paul probably meant, since that's the only perspective he had on food.

Did Paul have any idea that food could have a direct effect on our health?" No, he simply knew that you had to eat. Two thousand years ago, there was no concept that the *quality* of the food you ate affected the quality of the life that you lived.

When people got hungry, they ate something to fill their stomach. It didn't matter whether it was bread, rice, meat, milk, fruits, or vegetables. The protein or salt content of a food meant nothing to them.

As a Christian, you are spiritually free to eat whatever you want. Your salvation is not threatened just because you eat pig—but there may be negative consequences from a physical standpoint. Just because you are free to eat whatever you want, however, doesn't mean that you should. " 'Everything is permissible'—but not everything is beneficial. 'Everything is permissible'—but not everything is constructive." (1 Corinthians 10:23).

By the way, when Paul said "everything is permissible" he wasn't endorsing that concept, he was just *quoting* the very worldly, carnal Corinthians. He was taking their loose use of Christian liberty and qualifying it. It wasn't Paul that was saying that everything is permissible.

In Romans 14:20 Paul said, "Do not destroy the work of God for the sake of food. All food is clean." Even though we have freedom as Christians, Paul was saying in this chapter that we shouldn't abuse that freedom if it can potentially harm the faith of a new fellow believer. Once again, I believe he was saying that all food is spiritually clean. He was making the point, however, that our higher concern should be the benefit of our brothers and sisters in Christ even if it means partially limiting our own rights and freedoms. We are to love our neighbor as ourself.

- **But Jesus Said Not to Worry about What We Eat. Matthew 6:25–27** says:
  Therefore I tell you, do not worry about your life, what you will eat or drink; or about your body, what you will wear. Is not life more important than food, and the body more important than clothes? Look at the birds of the air; they do not sow or reap or store away in barns, and yet your heavenly Father feeds them. Are you not much more valuable than they? Who of you by worrying can add a single hour to his life?

Obviously, the point of this passage is not to be unconcerned about nutrition, but rather to avoid worry and anxiety. Jesus wants you to know that if God feeds the birds of the air and clothes the lilies, He certainly will take care of you.

- **Your Body, His Temple.**
  Paul said in **2 Corinthians 6:16**, "For we are the temple of the living God." Today, many people take better care of their cars than they do this temple of the Holy Spirit. They regularly change the oil, get a tune-up, and rotate the

tires on their cars. They wash, wax, and do everything they can to make their cars look like new. Unfortunately, the ashtray is often full of cigarette butts, and the seat is pushed all the way back to accommodate an ever-increasing waistline.

Some might say, "It's my body, I can do what I want to." But you know as a Christian that it's *not* your body. 1 Corinthians 6:19 tells us:

> Do you not know that your body is a temple of the Holy Spirit, who is in you, whom you have received from God? You are not your own; you were bought with a price. Therefore honor God with your body.

You are an incredible creation of God according to Psalm 139:13–14: "For you created my inmost being; you knit me together in my mother's womb. I praise you because I am fearfully and wonderfully made."

"But," some would ask, "shouldn't we be spending our time reading the Bible and developing our mind and spirit on the things of God? It's not good to get so obsessed with your body."

First of all, obsession with their body and health is *not* a problem with most Christians. Avoidance of the issue *is*. Many can quote lots of Bible verses, but they have no idea of their current HDL level. It's good, of course, to know lots of Bible verses, but we should at least also know the basics of temple maintenance too.

Second, investing time in the physical health of your body is *not* being too secular. The view that our physical body is somehow not worthy of our time compared to the importance of our spiritual life comes from ancient Greek philosophy, not from the Bible.

Paul said in 1 Timothy 4:8, "For physical training is of some value, but godliness has value for all things, holding promise for both the present life and the life to come." He did not say that physical health is useless. He simply compared physical health to the eternal benefits of spiritual health. And, of course, that's correct.

But we're not faced here with an either/or situation. You can be *both* physically and spiritually healthy at the same time. Indeed, it's been my experience that when I feel good *physically*, I feel better *spiritually* too.

Jesus valued physical health as well. In example after example (Mark 6:5; Luke 5:17; Luke 7:3; John 11:43), Jesus acknowledged through His healing ministry that the physical and health needs of people were important. He could have simply said "your sins are forgiven" and sent them on their way. He chose, instead, to demonstrate His love by also addressing the immediate needs of their physical health as well.

In John 2:19 Jesus also called *His* body a temple. In 1 Corinthians 3:16 Paul says, "Don't you know that you yourselves are God's temple. . . . If anyone destroys God's temple, God will destroy him." Is it any wonder that people who smoke cigarettes for 40 years get cancer?

Does the New Testament tell us that God's dietary laws no longer apply? A closer look at Scripture would suggest that, indeed, the opposite may be true. When we read the Bible in the context in which it was written, it's clear that modern-day Christians might need to take a serious second look at God's dietary laws.

Hilkiah the high priest said to Shapan the secretary, 'I have found the Book of the Law...' And Shapan read from it in the presence of the king. When the king heard the words of the Book of the Law, he tore his robes. [because he realized how far the nation had strayed from God's commands]
2 Kings 22: 8, 11

30

Did Jesus Eat Ham on Easter Sunday?

D id Jesus ever break the dietary laws? If He did, that would settle the issue for us today. Consider Luke 24:41–43. After the resurrection, the first thing Jesus did after revealing Himself to His disciples was to ask, "Do you have anything here to eat?" They gave Him a piece of broiled fish, and He took it and ate it in their presence. We also know Jesus ate bread and drank wine at the Last Supper (Mark 14:22–25). Yet we have no evidence that Jesus broke the dietary laws.

Jesus certainly had the opportunity to break the dietary laws during his three-year ministry. He certainly took the opportunity of his ministry to correct misconceptions in other areas. He *made a point* of breaking the Jewish traditions.

Jesus associated and ate with sinners (Matthew 9:10). He allowed His disciples to glean wheat on the Sabbath (Matthew

12:1) and He healed on the Sabbath too (John 5:9-16 and John 9:14). He drove the money changers out of the temple (Mark 11:15) and basically pointed out the barrenness and hypocrisy of the Jewish traditions.

Jesus put things in perspective. Yet He made it clear that God's Law was still the standard. In Matthew 23:23 Jesus said:

> Woe to you, teachers of the law and Pharisees, you hypocrites! You give a tenth of your spices—mint, dill and cumin. But you have neglected *the more important matters* of the law—justice, mercy and faithfulness. You should have practiced the latter, *without neglecting the former*. You blind guides! You strain out a gnat but swallow a camel.

When Jesus healed the leper in Matthew 8:3–4 He told him, "But go, show yourself to the priest and offer the gift Moses commanded, as a testimony to them." Here Jesus had a perfect opportunity to do away with the old law but instead He encouraged the healed leper to honor it nevertheless. In Matthew 5:17 Jesus said, "Do not think that I have come to abolish the Law or the Prophets; I have not come to abolish them but to fulfill them."

The account of the demon-possessed man is given in Mark 5:1–17. Chains couldn't bind him, and no one was strong enough to subdue him. Jesus commanded that the demons leave him, and He sent them into a herd of cattle on the hill. Is that correct? No, he sent them into a herd of pigs. The pigs then ran down the hill and into the water and were drowned. Could Jesus have been giving us a subtle message that those pigs weren't of much value anyway? Isn't it ironic that on Easter—the day we celebrate Jesus' resurrection—many Christians eat ham, a food that Jesus may never have eaten Himself.

As far as we can tell, Jesus never broke the dietary laws.

31

God's Dietary Guidelines

You already know, from Chapter 27, the official Dietary Guidelines for Americans. But what, specifically, does *God* say about the food we eat?

Fruits and Vegetables

Let's begin with Genesis 1:29–30:

> I give you every seed-bearing plant on the face of the whole earth and every tree that has fruit with seed in it. They will be yours for food. And to all the beasts of the earth and all the birds of the air and all the creatures that move on the ground—everything that has the breath of life in it—I give every green plant for food.

It appears that we were all originally vegetarians! But don't worry. You don't have to give up hamburgers. As you'll see, beef is okay.

If you have a steak, however, you may want to leave the mushrooms off. A mushroom is a fungus, not a plant. It reproduces through spores, not seeds. Another fungus, mildew, is specifically spoken against in Leviticus 13 and 14. You may like mushrooms, but you may want to reconsider whether or not they should be on your plate.

Meat

It wasn't until after the flood that God added meat to our menu. Genesis 9:3 says, "Everything that lives and moves will be food for you. Just as I gave you the green plants, I now give you everything." It's my opinion that the "everything" did not include the unclean animals that God had already identified before the flood. The point is that God was now also allowing meat for food. As we've said earlier, it's animal *fat* that God doesn't want us to eat. As far as what is acceptable, the details can be found in Deuteronomy 14:4–21 and Leviticus 11.

> For everything that was written in the past was written to teach us, so that through endurance and the encouragement of the Scriptures we might have hope.
> *Romans 15:4*

Specifically, Deuteronomy 14:6 says,

> You may eat any animal that has a split hoof divided in two and that chews the cud.

A cow, for example, chews its cud and has a split hoof. Beef, therefore, is acceptable— not fatty beef, but lean beef. On the other hand, a camel chews its cud but doesn't have a split hoof. Camel, therefore, is unclean. How about a pig? It has a split hoof, but it doesn't chew its cud. Therefore, according to God's

Word, you'd probably be better off not eating pig.

Some people might argue that the dietary laws prohibited unclean animals because they were unsafe to eat in biblical times. Today it's different, they say, because pigs are raised in

> The average American eats about 50 pounds of pig a year.

modern sanitary conditions and fed a good diet. It is actually true that pigs are leaner today than ever before. Not only are farmers raising leaner pigs, but butchers are cutting off more fat from the meat as well.

But if one agrees with that line of thinking, the question then becomes *when* did pig become acceptable to consume? The Scripture doesn't say pigs are unclean until they can be raised in sanitary conditions. Is there a time limitation on God's wisdom? What if there's something about the very physiology of the pig that makes it bad for human consumption? What if science doesn't discover what it is until 20 years from now?

If Jesus' resurrection did away with the dietary laws, that must mean that pigs automatically became clean as soon as He was resurrected. Did the very physical nature of pigs change that first Easter morning? No.

The only argument that can be made here is that the unclean foods were merely symbolically unclean. But with that line of thinking we must also acknowledge that the laws regarding circumcision, avoidance of animal fat, and other issues all were simply symbolic also, having no real physical world benefits.

We've already established that God's law *does* benefit us in both the spiritual and *physical* realms. Pigs are just as physically unclean by nature today as they were 2,000 years ago. You can't make a silk purse out of a pig's ear—regardless of how sanitary the conditions are.

Seafood

Deuteronomy 14:9 says, "Of all the creatures living in the water, you may eat any that has fins and scales." According to God's Word, therefore, catfish is not acceptable. A catfish has fins but no scales—its skin is smooth. It's unclean.

A lot of catfish is now farm raised. They're grain fed as well. You could certainly make a case that these are improvements over catfish that you'd catch in a pond. Once again, however, Scripture doesn't reveal any conditions under which catfish can become clean.

Referring to the fishermen's net, Jesus said, "When it was full, the fishermen pulled it up on the shore. Then they sat down and collected the good fish in baskets, but threw the bad away" (Matthew 13:48). What could the bad fish be? Possibly dead fish. The possibility also exists that Jesus was still acknowledging the dietary laws by stating the obvious-at-that-time fact that some fish are unacceptable.

Science has now shown that shellfish are a nutritionally acceptable food. With 200 mg of cholesterol in a 3.5 ounce serving, shrimp, for example, is still high in cholesterol, but it's extremely low in the bad saturated fat.

Shellfish also contain the good omega-3 fats. As a result, the American Heart Association, along with other health organizations that formerly discouraged shellfish, have now acknowledged that, indeed, shellfish can be a part of a heart-healthy diet.

But what does the Bible say? Do shellfish have scales? No. Fins? No. According to God's Word, then, you may be better off not eating shellfish. "You mean I *have to* give up lobster and shrimp?" No, but you may want to anyway.

Birds

Birds are listed in Deuteronomy 14:11–18:

> You may eat any clean bird. But these you may not eat: the eagle, the vulture, the black vulture, the red kite, the black kite, any kind of falcon, any kind of raven, the horned owl, the screech owl, the gull, any kind of hawk, the little owl, the great owl, the white owl, the desert owl, the osprey, the cormorant, the stork, any kind of heron, the hoopoe and the bat.

Fortunately, most of these birds aren't on your Top 10 Favorites list. By listing only the unclean birds, God identified all others as clean simply by their absence from the list. Chicken is, therefore, okay. Hooray!

God, speaking of the evil princes of Jerusalem: "They teach that there is no difference between the unclean and the clean."
Ezekiel 22:26

Figure 31.1

CLEAN AND UNCLEAN FOOD
(American Culture)

CLEAN

Beef	Vegetable fat[1]	Grouper	Sardine
Buffalo	Fish[2]	Haddock	Smelt
Chicken	Anchovy	Halibut	Snapper
Deer/Venison	Barracuda	Herring	Sole
Duck	Bass	Mackerel[4]	Spot
Elk	Bonito	Orange roughy	Trout
Goat	Carp	Perch	Tuna
Goose	Cod	Pike	Walleye
Moose	Dolphin fish	Pollock	Whitefish
Sheep/Lamb	or mahimahi[3]	Rockfish	Whiting
Turkey	Flounder	Salmon	

1. Any oil or fat that comes from a plant is clean. Olive oil, canola oil, peanut oil, corn oil, safflower oil, soybean oil, cottonseed oil, etc., mayonnaise, margarine.
2. Almost all fish you are familiar with are clean. The more common unclean fish are listed in the box below.
3. Note: dolphins, porpoises, and whales are mammals, not fish, and therefore not clean.
4. All except snake mackerel.

UNCLEAN

Animal fat (butter, lard, visible meat fat, cream)[1]	Lobster	Eel	Sailfish
	Mussels	Firefish	Sculpin
	Oysters	Gar	Shark[3]
Frog	Scallops	Goosefish	Snake mackerel
Gelatin[2]	Shrimp	Lamprey	
Mushrooms	Snail	Leatherjacket	Sturgeon[3]
Pig	Snake	Lomosucker	Swordfish[3]
Possum	Squirrel	Marlin	Toadfish
Rabbit	Fish	Ocean pout	Triggerfish
Seafood	Billfish	Oilfish	Trunkfish
Clams	Catfish	Puffer	Wolffish
Crab	Cutlassfish	Rock prickleback	

1. The Bible specifically talks about animal fat as being unacceptable for human consumption. In the context of what was being written it's literally talking about visible animal fat. I'm *adding* butter, lard, and cream to that list too since they are all, in fact, animal fat as well. Today we know that animal fat is saturated fat—and it doesn't matter whether it comes from visible meat fat, butter, lard, or cream—none of it is good for your health. Now it could be argued that if the Bible only identifies visible meat fat as unclean, then that's all we should put on the list. If you want to look at it that way, that's fine. But I'm going to take the position that these fats are just another form of visible animal fat.
2. Gelatin is made from the hide trimmings of cows and pigs.
3. Jewish tradition counts these as unclean because of their unusual kind of "scales."

What Was God Thinking?

Could there be some logical reason for identifying certain foods as unclean? Or did God just randomly choose certain creatures to be off-limits? Was God's intention one of establishing obedience and distinguishing the nation of Israel from all others, or might there also be a more practical reason to avoid these particular foods?

Why would God tell us *not* to eat something as tasty as lobster and shrimp? Do these unclean foods have something in common that might help explain this prohibition?

Almost all of the creatures on the unclean list are scavengers. In many cases they don't hunt for their own food; they eat the dead and decaying matter of our environment. A catfish does that at the bottom of a pond; lobsters and shrimp do it in the ocean. A pig will eat anything. Vultures, almost by definition, are known for their scavenger habits.

Could it be that God, in His wisdom, created certain creatures whose sole purpose is to clean up after the others? Their entire "calling" may be to act exclusively as the sanitation workers of our ecology. God may simply be telling us that it's better for us believers not to consume the meat of these trash collectors.

> Even more important than whether the Old Testament dietary laws apply to Christians today, may be the issue of whether we have to completely figure out God's Word before we consider obeying it.

Even more important than whether the Old Testament dietary laws apply to Christians today, may be the issue of whether we have to completely figure out God's Word before we consider obeying it. Do God's directives have to make logical sense to our limited minds before we're willing to try them?

God said in Isaiah 55:8, "My thoughts are not your thoughts, neither are your ways my ways." In Mark 10:15 we read, "I tell you the truth, anyone who will not receive the kingdom of God like a little child will never enter it." God wants us to trust His Word.

Much of the wisdom revealed in the Bible now makes sense to us from our modern perspective, but should that mean we won't consider the areas that haven't yet been scientifically proven? We've only discovered that animal fat is bad for us in the last 50 years. To the Christian a century ago, the directive in Leviticus 3:17 to avoid animal fat made no sense at all. Yet it's clear to us today. What if there's something in lobster that's harmful to our health? What if we don't discover what it is until 50 years from now? Do we require scientific proof before we give the Bible the benefit of the doubt?

No, We're Not Talking Kosher

Would God have us eat like the Orthodox Jews? I don't think so. Exodus 23:19, Exodus 34:26, and Deuteronomy 14:21 all say, "Do not cook a young goat in its mother's milk." Between me and you, I don't personally cook that much goat anymore! Nevertheless, God says don't do it. Don't take a baby goat and boil it in its mother's milk. That's clear enough.

With all good intentions, over the years, the Jewish tradition has built up fences around God's laws so that no one could ever get close to breaking them. Good intentions aside, it's important that we follow God's Word, not man's expansion of that Word. Orthodox kosher observance has now gone so far as to require a person to never eat *any* meat product and *any* dairy product at the same time. It even requires separate sets of dinnerware and flatware—one for dairy products, one for meat products. You're not even supposed to use the same dishwater when you wash the dishes!

Those are human rules. God's Word simply states, "Do not cook a young goat in its mother's milk." So while we agree on the specific biblical dietary guidelines, we're not embracing the legalism of kosher eating that we see in Orthodox Judaism today. What we *are* doing is taking advantage of God's time-less wisdom, as revealed in the Bible.

But Why Do They Taste So Good?

Frankly, I like the taste of pork chops, shrimp, lobster, and ham. I like fried catfish too! But I choose not to eat them any-more. In His dietary laws, God is not trying to take away foods that give us pleasure. He is, in reality, *trying to build our faith!* What kind of obedience would it take if He prohib-ited foods that tasted *bad*? None!

Did it ever occur to you that God could quite easily have made every single food on earth *good* for you? God could have made *everything* taste as good as ice cream and be as nutritious as broccoli. But He didn't.

> God could have made *everything* taste as good as ice cream and be as nutritious as broccoli.

God may have designated cer-tain foods as unclean as part of His bigger plan to simply build your faith. He wants your trust and obedience in Him to mature. He wants us to get to the point where we have *complete* confidence that His ways are sometimes beyond our understanding.

God sure puts a lot of emphasis on building our trust in Him. He must have some mighty important work waiting for us when we get to heaven!

32

Does This
Work?

C an you expect to see some benefits from following the Old
  Testament dietary laws? Is it worth the effort? Consider
the first chapter of Daniel:

> In the third year of the reign of Jehoiakim king of
> Judah, Nebuchadnezzar king of Babylon came to Jerusa-
> lem and besieged it. And the Lord delivered Jehoiakim
> King of Judah into his hand, along with some of the arti-
> cles from the temple of God. These he carried off to the
> temple of his god in Babylonia and put in the treasure
> house of his god.
>
> Then the king ordered Ashpenaz, chief of his court
> officials, to bring in some of the Israelites from the
> royal family and the nobility—young men without any
> physical defect, handsome, showing aptitude for every
> kind of learning, well informed, quick to understand,
> and qualified to serve in the king's palace. He was to

teach them the language and literature of the Babylonians. The king assigned them a daily amount of food and wine from the king's table. They were to be trained for three years, and after that they were to enter the king's service.

Among these were some from Judah: Daniel, Hananiah, Mishael and Azariah. The chief official gave them new names: to Daniel, the name Belteshazzar; to Hananiah, Shadrach; to Mishael, Meshach; and to Azariah, Abednego.

But Daniel resolved not to defile himself with the royal food and wine, and he asked the chief official for permission not to defile himself this way. Now God had caused the official to show favor and sympathy to Daniel, but the official told Daniel, "I am afraid of my lord the king, who has assigned your food and drink. Why should he see you looking worse than the other young men your age? The king would then have my head because of you."

Daniel then said to the guard whom the chief official had appointed over Daniel, Hananiah, Mishael and Azariah, "Please test your servants for ten days: Give us nothing but vegetables to eat and water to drink. Then compare our appearance with that of the young men who eat the royal food, and treat your servants in accordance with what you see." So he agreed to this and tested them for ten days.

At the end of the ten days they looked healthier and better nourished than any of the young men who ate the royal food. So the guard took away their choice food and the wine they were to drink and gave them vegetables instead.

To these four young men God gave knowledge and understanding of all kinds of literature and learning. And Daniel could understand visions and dreams of all kinds.

At the end of the time set by the king to bring them in, the chief official presented them to Nebuchadnezzar. The king talked to them, and he found none equal to Daniel, Hananiah, Mishael, and Azariah; so they entered the king's service. In every matter of wisdom and understanding about which the king questioned them, he found them ten times better than all the magicians and enchanters in his whole kingdom. And Daniel remained there until the first year of King Cyrus.

In the eighth verse Daniel resolves not to defile himself with the royal food and wine. Obviously, some of the food on the king's table must have been unclean by God's standards. What else could cause Daniel to be defiled? When he made arrangements to demonstrate the wisdom of God's Word, the results were clear. Again, Daniel 1:15 says, "At the end of the ten days they looked healthier and better nourished than any of the young men who ate the royal food."

The King James Version reads, "And at the end of ten days their countenances appeared fairer and fatter in flesh than all the children which did eat the portion of the king's meat." That's potentially confusing. Today, the last thing most of us want is to *get fatter!*

> # God's Word isn't going to make you gain weight.

No need to worry. God's Word isn't going to make you gain weight. The word translated *fatter* in the King James is the Hebrew word *tov*, meaning "good." It's the same word that is used in Genesis 1:4, "God saw that the light was *tov* ('good')."

In 1 Samuel 8:16 *tov* refers to well-nourished, well-built, strong beasts of burden. When the King James Version was translated in the 1600s, having extra fat on your body helped you survive when you couldn't eat because of an illness or disease. Skinny people were the ones who died first. Today with modern medicine and an emphasis on prevention, it's the obese people who are at higher risk.

The New International Version, in which Daniel and his colleagues are described as "healthier and better nourished," is more accurate. The point of the first chapter of Daniel is that God honored Daniel's decision to be obedient to the Word. If you follow what has been revealed through the Bible, should you expect any less from God?

> **God honored Daniel's decision to be obedient to the Word.**

Well, does this work *today*? I'm not promoting any particular theology here, but you may be familiar with the Seventh-day Adventists, who worship on Saturday instead of Sunday. They also choose to abstain from cigarettes and alcohol and more closely follow the biblical dietary guidelines of avoiding pig and shellfish and decreasing their intake of animal fat. The proof seems to be in the pudding.

Seventh-day Adventists have significantly less heart disease, strokes, and cancer compared to the average American! They've cut their risk of these diseases, for the most part, by simply applying God's Word to their life. If they can do it, why can't the rest of us?

What if all Christians started living years longer than their neighbors did? Would that make an impression on an unsaved world? Would that get their attention?

What if 70- and 80-year-old Christian men were still vibrant and full of life? What if they didn't die from stroke and heart disease like everyone else? In Deuteronomy 34:7 we see that Moses lived to 120, yet his eyesight was perfect and he was as strong as a young man.

What if Christian women didn't get uterine and breast cancer? What if diabetes were rare in those who acknowledged Jesus Christ as Lord? *That* would get the world's attention.

An unbelieving world would have to stop and ask, "What is going on with these people who call themselves Christians? What do *they* know that we don't? Just what's *in* that Bible that they read?" What a powerful witness that would be!

Hosea 4:6 says, "My people are destroyed from lack of knowledge." If Satan can't get someone to renounce Jesus Christ, and if he can't get them to stop proclaiming and evangelizing the simple message of salvation, isn't it just like him to sneak in the back door and cut that person's life off early?

Yes, God's people will go to heaven, but their ministry here, their time with their families, their productive years for the kingdom, might be cut terribly short—not from a mistake on their part, but simply from a lack of knowledge.

Jesus said we are truly His disciples when we follow His teachings. "Then you will know the truth, and the truth will set you free" (John 8:32).

> **M**y people are destroyed from lack of knowledge.
> *Hosea 4:6*

Yes You Can!

As I speak at churches and organizations all over the U.S. and Canada, I am continually amazed that some people completely turn their lives around after hearing a single speech. They dramatically improve their diet, get more physical activity, and really get serious about this temple that is so fearfully and wonderfully made.

And yet I'm equally amazed when others hear the same message, presented by the same speaker, in the same way, and walk out unchanged. They don't even try. Why is that?

To a large extent, I feel it's because many believers today don't really realize who they *are* as Christians. A healthy, Christ-centered self-esteem is not pompous or prideful. As a Christian, you *are* somebody! Not because of who *you* say you are, but because of who the *Creator of the universe* says you are!

When you truly understand the identity that Jehovah God has declared for you, everything changes! Suddenly you're somebody special. God knew you before you were ever born into this world (Jeremiah 1:5, Psalm 139:13). Listen to what *He* says about who *you* are:

- **A New Creation**: "Therefore, if anyone is in Christ, he is a new creation; the old has gone, the new has come!" (2 Corinthians 5:17).

- **An Instrument for Noble Purposes**: "He will be an instrument for noble purposes, made holy, useful to the Master and prepared to do any good work" (2 Timothy 2:21).

- **Victorious**: "But thanks be to God! He gives us the victory through our Lord Jesus Christ" (1 Corinthians 15:57).

- **Empowered by God**: "Now to him who is able to do immeasurably more than all we ask or imagine, according to his power that is at work within us" (Ephesians 3:20).

- **A Chosen People**: "But you are a chosen people, a royal priesthood, a holy nation, a people belonging to God" (1 Peter 2:9).

- **Clothed with Christ**: "For all of you who were baptized into Christ have clothed yourselves with Christ" (Galatians 3:27).

- **God's Treasured Possession**: "Out of all the peoples on the face of the earth, the LORD has chosen you to be his treasured possession" (Deuteronomy 14:2).

- **Loved by God for All of Eternity**: "For God so loved the world that he gave his one and only Son, that whoever believes in him shall not perish but have eternal life" (John 3:16).

If we believe that the Bible is God's revealed truth, why do so many Christians have such a poor outlook? "I can't lose weight." "I can't exercise regularly." "I can't stop smoking." "I've failed in the past, I'll just fail again." No wonder people who are exposed to the truth still don't take action. With that viewpoint, who would?

But *you* are different. You are a son or daughter of the almighty, living God! You have a reason to be here. You matter. You make a difference. Isn't it worth the effort to be all God wants you to be?

The Bible says that someday you will have an opportunity to present your life before Christ. Will it be one of excuses or one of joyous service? Having great health can help make that positive life a real possibility. As a Christian you *are* somebody. Act like it!

Just Do It

What if you could be absolutely convinced that the Old Testament dietary laws apply to you today? Would you follow them then?

What proof do you need? How about hearing from God Himself? Would *that* do it?

Isn't the Bible hearing from God Himself? Isn't that what we Christians profess? *When has God's Word ever let you down?* Has the Bible ever steered you down the wrong path? Have you ever been disappointed by the revealed truth of God? Can you think of a situation where you couldn't trust God's Word as the ultimate authority for an important decision in your life? Are you willing to at least give God the benefit of the doubt?

When I was a young boy and my dad told me not to play out in the street, I had two choices.

I could choose *not* to listen. I could have said, "It's fun to play out in the street. He just doesn't want me to have any fun. Besides, other kids play in the street. Why can't I?" I could have disregarded years of good counsel and protection. Eventually, a car could have hit me.

On the other hand, I could have simply trusted my dad. I could have said, "He's always treated me well. He puts a roof over my head, gives me food to eat, and takes me to the doctor when I get sick. There's no reason I shouldn't trust him at this point. After all, he didn't tell me I couldn't play—he just said to play in the safety of the yard. If he says I'm better off staying out of the street, I'll take him at his word." With that attitude I never would have been in danger.

I believe that God tells us through the Bible that He has created the entire bounty of the world's food for us to consume. He created several living things for other purposes, however, and they're not for consumption as food. You'll be better off not eating them.

> This is love for God: to obey his commands.
> And his commands are not burdensome.
> *1 John 5:3*

God isn't trying to impose some burdensome restrictions on you. It's just that He knows how the human body works—after all, He created it! God is the author of human life, and through the Bible He's given you the owner's manual.

If an owner's manual for a 1931 car was good for that automobile in 1931, then it's still good for that automobile today. The physiology and anatomy of our bodies hasn't changed in the short time since Scripture was written. If it was good for God's people then, it's probably still good for God's people now.

Your decision to follow God's dietary guidelines really comes down to a matter of faith. Isn't God's Word enough? Are you willing to let your taste buds make a spiritual decision for you?

This may, in fact, also be a matter of sanctification—a

matter of spiritual maturity—not necessarily based on *what* you decide, but on whether you will at least seriously consider it.

If for no other reason, the biblical dietary laws are worthy of your consideration just because God said it.

Practices like circumcision and the avoidance of animal fat didn't make much sense to God's people originally. But they nevertheless received benefit from following His guidelines anyway.

This is really more than just an issue of what to eat and what not to eat. It's an issue of trusting God. Keep in mind that God gave Adam and Eve all of the trees of the garden for food, but He set limits. He told them to eat anything they wanted except for the fruit of one particular tree. He warned there would be consequences, yet the fruit was "good for food and pleasing to the eye" (Genesis 3:6). If they would have only chosen to obey God's original dietary command!

Will *you* choose to obey God's dietary laws? I believe that if you combine the wisdom of the Bible with what you've learned here about good health, you can look forward to a better life even *before* you get to heaven. May God bless you in your efforts.

ACTION STEPS
FOR EATING BY THE BOOK

1. Prayerfully ask God for His insight regarding the dietary laws.

2. Read and study the cited Scriptures for yourself.

3. Remember that you don't *have to* follow the dietary laws—but you may want to, nevertheless.

4. If you believe that God's dietary laws still have merit today, refer to page 228 for the particular foods that God has identified as best for you.

5. Rejoice in the fact that you serve a God who doesn't demand that you follow a long list of rules to become "good enough" to please Him. Thank Him that Jesus Christ is all you need for salvation. But also thank Him for the timeless, practical wisdom of His Word, which benefits us today as much as it did when it was written thousands of years ago.

AFTERWORD

A Final Thought

Thank you for making it all the way through what I hope was a great learning experience for you.

Obviously, this book was written with the Christian in mind. The scientific and factual matter of this work, however, is applicable to you regardless of where you are in your spiritual journey.

It's my hope that as a result of what you've learned here you can experience greater, more vibrant health than ever before. You may ultimately end up running marathons, memorizing every nutrition label in your grocery store, and attaining the ideal body fat percentage. The unfortunate reality remains, however, that finally, some day, some way, you will still have to die. The mortality rate of we humans remains 100 percent. No one has got out alive yet. You have tremendous control over the quantity and quality of your life, but what you don't have control over is your ultimate mortality.

You've heard of people who were in the very best of health being quickly struck down by a fast spreading cancer. You may also know of someone who was at the top of the world suddenly killed in an accident by a drunk driver. At home with the family one evening, dead the next. The reality is that we are all just one heartbeat away from eternity.

The Christian faith is based on several presuppositions: that God does exist, that we can know Him through the Bible, and that we will all spend eternity somewhere. The Bible also tells us that we will all someday face God to give an accounting of our life.

If you were to die tonight, do you know *for certain* that you would go to heaven? If you're not absolutely sure, the Bible tells you how you can be. If you were to face God tonight and He asked you why you should be allowed into heaven, what would you say? Would you claim that you were a decent, nice person? After all, you've never killed anyone or committed any major crime. Besides, you've been a good parent, a loyal employee, and certainly a much better person than a lot of other people you know. If your answer to God would be something along these lines, you may be very surprised to see what the Bible says about all your good deeds. Just as you've learned about your physical health, I now want to encourage you to learn about your spiritual health.

I'm amazed at the number of people who have very definite opinions about the Bible but have never read the whole book. It took me several years, but I ultimately accomplished that goal. In the process I was surprised to learn how relevant Scripture is to the science of health. The book you're holding is a result of that discovery. I think you'll be amazed to see how relevant God's Word is to your personal life today, as well. If you've been intimidated by the complexity of bibles you've seen in the past, now there's good news. There are several new versions of the Bible that are written in today's American language that you *can* understand. I'd suggest you start with *The Message* or *The New Living Translation,* both of which are available at your local bookstore.

If you don't have the assurance that you know absolutely that you'll spend eternity in heaven, I'd be honored to help you discover how you can have that assurance.

If you'll write to me, I'll be glad to send at no cost some literature that explains what the Bible says about God and your relationship with Him. Incidentally, the news is *very* good.

I wish you the very best of both physical and spiritual health.

David Meinz

PO Box 772525, Orlando, FL 32877

www.DavidMeinz.com

APPENDIX I

Canadian Recommended Blood Cholesterol Levels

The new Canadian guidelines emphasize a more aggressive approach to lowering LDL ("bad" cholesterol) levels in relation to HDL ("good" cholesterol) levels and recommend that people at high risk – for example, those with a history of heart disease, or diabetes – be treated with lipid-lowering drugs immediately, along with any necessary lifestyle changes *to achieve the following recommended targets*:

THOSE AT HIGH RISK

LDL Level . . . . *less than* 2.5 mmol/L
Ratio of Total Cholesterol to HDL . . . . *less than* 4.0

THOSE AT MODERATE RISK

LDL Level . . . . *less than* 3.5 mmol/L
Ratio of Total Cholesterol to HDL . . . . *less than* 5.0

THOSE AT LOW RISK

LDL level . . . . *less than* 4.5 mmol/L
Ratio of Total Cholesterol to HDL . . . . *less than* 6.0

- To convert a Canadian measure to U.S. measures, multiply the Canadian number by 38.7 (you can round it off to 40 to make it easier, if you wish). For example, 0.9 mmol/L in Canadian measures is about 34.8 mg/dL (or approximately 35) in U.S. units.

- Conversely, if you want to convert a U.S. measurement to the Canadian equivalent, divide the amount in mg/dL by 38.7. For example, 200 mg/dL divided by 38.7 is 5.2 mmol/L.

APPENDIX II

Modifying Recipes and Menus to Meet the Dietary Guidelines for Americans

By carefully purchasing foods, preparing foods in different ways or substituting ingredients, diets can be made healthier. On the following pages, suggestions for reducing the fat, sodium and sugar, and increasing the amount of fiber in recipes are provided. Remember, diets of children less than two years of age should not be restrictive.

When purchasing foods, compare the ingredient lists and nutrition panels on labels of several brands of a food product. Select the brand that contains the least amount of fat, sodium and sugar, and the greatest amount of fiber.

When modifying recipes, make one modification in a recipe at a time. Reduce or increase the amount of the ingredient to be modified by a small amount at first. Try additional modifications in the recipe later.

Baked products require more careful adjustments than casseroles or soups. For example, drastically reducing the amount of sugar in a cake or fat in biscuits may result in unsatisfactory products. A reduction in fat or sugar may require a slight increase in the amount of liquid used.

Every ingredient has an important role in the production of a satisfactory final product.

- **Fat**
  Fat provides flavor and richness, improves texture, tenderness, flakiness, and lightness in baked goods, and makes foods smooth and creamy.

- **Eggs**
  Eggs provide structure, act as thickeners and emulsifiers (help mix fat and water), and add volume to foods when beaten.

- **Sugar**
  Sugar provides flavor, increases tenderness and browning in baked goods, acts as a preservative in jams, jellies and pickles, and helps yeast products rise.

- **Salt**
  Salt provides flavor, slows or reduces the action of yeast in yeast breads, and acts as a preservative in canned goods and some dried foods.

Suggestions for Reducing Fat

- Use low-fat (1%) or fat free milk rather than whole milk or reduced-fat milk.
- Replace sour cream with low-fat yogurt. Add one tablespoon of cornstarch to every one cup of yogurt to prevent separation when heating.
- Blend mayonnaise with low-fat cottage cheese for a low-fat mayonnaise substitute or purchase commercial low-fat mayonnaise.
- Purchase water-packed tuna rather than oil-packed tuna.
- Use low-fat varieties of cheese such as part-skim mozzarella, farmer cheese, muenster, provolone, reduced-fat cheddar, or American cheese.
- Choose ground beef that is at least 85% lean (less than 15% fat).
- Substitute lean ground turkey for all or part of ground beef in recipes.
- Remove skin from poultry and trim off fat.
- Chill soups, gravies, and stews. Skim off hardened fat before reheating to serve.
- Trim off all visible fat from meats.
- Drain all fat from cooked meats.
- Substitute two egg whites for each whole egg in most muffin, cookie, or pudding recipes.
- Use buttermilk or milk instead of egg to bind breading on chicken.
- Use half the specified amount of oil to saute or brown foods.
- Substitute applesauce for one-half of the butter or margarine in cookies or cakes.
- Bake, broil, or roast rather than fry meat.
- Replace hot dogs, bologna, or other processed meat with lean meat, poultry, or fish.
- Limit the use of pan-fried or deep-fat-fried foods.
- Limit the use of high-fat crackers and breads such as croissants and some muffins and specialty breads.
- Garnish fish with lemon juice rather than tartar sauce.

Suggestions for Reducing Sugar

• Use up to one-third less sugar in traditional recipes for cookies, muffins, quick breads, and pie fillings. This includes sugar, brown sugar, corn syrup, honey and molasses.

• Replace canned fruits packed in heavy syrup with fresh fruits or canned fruits packed in natural juices or water.

• Limit the use of jams, jellies, or flavored gelatins.

• Serve quick breads rather than high sugar cakes or cookies. Try banana, carrot, cranberry, pumpkin, or zucchini bread.

• Serve seasonal fresh fruits for dessert rather than cakes, cookies, or pies.

Suggestions for Increasing Fiber

• Substitute whole wheat flour for up to one-half of the all-purpose flour in your favorite bread recipes.

• Substitute beans (kidney, pinto, or black) for up to one-half of the meat in entreés such as chili or tacos.

• Add fruits, such as chopped apples with skin, raisins, or chopped prunes, to oatmeal, cookies, cakes, and breads.

• Use oatmeal rather than white bread crumbs as an extender in meatloaf or meatballs.

• Serve raw vegetables, such as broccoli, cauliflower, carrots, and celery, for snacks.

• Top cereals with fresh or frozen fruits, such as blueberries, bananas, or peaches.

Suggestions for Reducing Sodium

- Omit or reduce by one-half the amount of salt in most recipes
- Include a variety of spices, seasonings, herbs, and vegetables in recipes rather than salt. For example, try chives, dill, garlic, or vinegar on cucumbers; serve green beans with lemon juice or sautéed onions; top potatoes with parsley; try bay leaf, onion, or thyme on beef; season poultry with lemon juice, marjoram, paprika, parsley, sage, or thyme; or season fish with bay leaf, curry powder, lemon juice, or paprika.
- Decrease the use of celery salt, seasoned salt, soy sauce, monosodium glutamate (MSG), Worcestershire sauce, or bouillon cubes
- Use garlic or onion powder in place of garlic or onion salt.
- Make soup stock from turkey, chicken, or beef bones, limiting the amount of bouillon added.
- Use fresh or frozen foods rather than canned foods.
- Serve processed meats only occasionally.

Healthful Ingredient Substitutions

You can increase nutrition and trim the fat in many of your favorite recipes easily and deliciously by using the substitutions listed below.

INSTEAD OF . . . | TRY:

INSTEAD OF . . .	TRY:
Salad dressing	Flavored vinegars (e.g. balsamic, raspberry); gourmet mustards; low-fat or non-fat dressing varieties
Iceberg lettuce	Spinach; romaine; other dark green leafy lettuces
Butter/margarine as spread	fat free/reduced fat margarine; liquid margarine; apple butter; preserves; jam
Cream cheese as spread	Neufchâtel cheese; light or nonfat cream cheese
Sour cream for dips	fat free ricotta; cottage cheese; fat free dips

INSTEAD OF . . .	TRY:
1 cup cream	1 cup evaporated fat free milk
Cream to thicken soups	Potato purée
Oil as base for marinade	Citrus juice; flavored vinegar
Oil or butter for sauté	Chicken or vegetable broth (as needed)
Chopped nuts	Water chestnuts; jicama
2 oz grated mild cheddar cheese	1 oz reduced fat sharp cheddar cheese
High fat sauces over meat/poultry	Vegetable purées (try steamed broccoli, meat/poultry sautéed onion, and garlic, salt and pepper to taste. Purée in food processor or blender.)
Ground beef	Ground turkey breast

INSTEAD OF . . .	TRY:
1 oz baking chocolate	3–4 tbsp cocoa powder + 1 tbsp oil (for frosting or sauces); $1/4$ cup cocoa (for cakes or cookies)
1 egg	2 egg whites; $1/4$ cup liquid egg substitute
$1/2$ cup butter/margarine	$1/4$ cup applesauce (or prune purée) + $1/4$ cup butter/margarine/oil
1 cup sour cream	1 cup nonfat or low-fat plain yogurt (if used in sauce, add 1 tbsp cornstarch)
Sweetened condensed milk	Low-fat/nonfat sweetened condensed milk
1 can evaporated milk	1 can evaporated fat free milk
1 cup all-purpose flour	1 cup finely milled whole wheat flour
Pie filling	Light fruit filling, low-fat pudding
Pastry pie crust	Graham cracker crust
1 cup chocolate chips	$1/2$ cup mini–chocolate chips
Sponge/pound cake	Angel food cake; fat free loaf cake
Fudge sauce	Chocolate syrup

Reprinted with permission of the American Institute for Cancer Research, Washington, D.C.

APPENDIX III

Clean and Healthy Recipes

It's been my observation that, for the most part, the majority of families eat the same ten or so recipes over and over. Here you'll find basic, popular, tasty recipes in much healthier versions.

Remember your "Rules of the Game," on page 195. Incidentally, don't be intimidated by sodium numbers here that sometimes may appear high. Keep in mind that you're easily allowed 2,000 mg of sodium a day. The point is, we've significantly reduced the fat and saturated fat and still maintained great flavor.

Regarding desserts, remember that reduced-fat and low-fat baked goods are often still high in calories because of their sugar content. Portion control is still necessary. You can top a dessert with fresh fruit to stretch the portion size and improve the presentation.

STUFFED FRENCH TOAST
serves 8

1 cup egg substitute
1/2 c skim milk
1 teaspoon vanilla
2 teaspoons cinnamon
8 slices whole wheat or raisin bread
1 (3 ounce) package nonfat cream cheese, softened
1/2 cup strawberry or raspberry preserves, or orange marmalade
Vegetable cooking spray
Confectioners sugar

In a medium bowl whisk together the egg substitute, skim milk, vanilla and cinnamon. Set aside.

In a separate medium bowl beat together the softened nonfat cream cheese with the preserves or marmalade. Spread the mixture evenly on the eight slices of bread and then sandwich the slices together. Dip a filled bread sandwich into the egg mixture coating on both sides.

Lightly spray a large nonstick skillet with vegetable spray and heat over medium heat. Place the dipped bread into a skillet and cook over medium heat until each side is golden brown, about 1 minute per side. Repeat with the remaining three dipped sandwiches using more vegetable spray in the skillet as needed.

Cut each sandwich in half diagonally and top with sliced peaches, bananas, or your choice of fresh fruit! Dust with Confectioners sugar and serve at once.

Nutrition Analysis
1/2 Sandwich

Stuffed French Toast	Traditional Stuffed French Toast
Fat 2g	Fat 15g
Saturated Fat 1g	Saturated Fat 7g
Sodium 607mg	Sodium 615mg
Cholesterol 57mg	Cholesterol 285mg
Calories 339	Calories 495

BEST OVEN "FRIED" CHICKEN
serves 6

1 cup egg substitute
1 cup skim milk
1/2 cup yellow cornmeal (not cornmeal mix)
1/2 cup reduced fat seasoned breadcrumbs
salt to taste
1 teaspoon black pepper
1 teaspoon poultry seasoning
1 teaspoon paprika
1 teaspoon garlic powder
1 teaspoon onion powder
1/2 teaspoon celery seed
2 cups crushed corn flake cereal
6 boneless, skinless chicken breasts

Preheat the oven to 400 degrees. Lightly coat a baking sheet with vegetable spray. Set aside.

In a small bowl combine the egg substitute and skim milk. In a shallow pie plate combine the cornmeal, breadcrumbs, salt, pepper, poultry seasoning, paprika, garlic powder, onion powder, and the celery seed. Place the crushed corn flake cereal in a second pie plate.

Dip one breast in the egg/milk mixture, then in the seasoned cornmeal, back into the egg/milk mixture and finally into the crushed corn flakes. Place on a wire rack and repeat the dipping procedure with the remaining breast. Place the chicken breasts on the prepared baking sheet and place in the preheated oven. Bake for 30–35 minutes or until the chicken breasts are crispy and golden brown. Serve at once.

Note: The proportions of the seasonings in the cornmeal mixture can be adjusted to suit your particular taste. Double dipping the breasts assures a crispy coat.

Nutrition Analysis
1 Chicken Breast

Best Oven "Fried" Chicken	Traditional Fried Chicken
Fat 5g	Fat 32g
Saturated Fat 1g	Saturated Fat 9g
Sodium 525mg	Sodium 682mg
Cholesterol 98mg	Cholesterol 210mg
Calories 330	Calories 644

CLASSIC MEATLOAF
serves 8

2 pounds ground turkey
1 onion, finely chopped
2 garlic cloves, finely chopped
4 green onions, finely chopped
4 egg whites, lightly beaten
1 cup reduced fat seasoned breadcrumbs
1 tablespoon dried Italian Seasoning
1 teaspoon ground cumin
1/4 cup freshly chopped parsley
1 1/2 cups jarred tomato or spaghetti sauce
salt and freshly ground black pepper to taste

Preheat the oven to 375 degrees. Lightly coat a medium baking pan with vegetable spray.

In a large bowl combine the ground turkey, onion, garlic, green onions, egg whites, breadcrumbs, cumin, dried Italian seasoning and salt and pepper to taste. Shape the mixture into a loaf and place in the prepared pan. Pour the jarred sauce over the meatloaf. Place in the oven and bake for one hour. Remove from the oven and allow to sit 10 minutes before slicing.

Nutrition Analysis
(7oz.)

Classic Meatloaf		Traditional Meat Loaf	
Fat	10g	Fat	21g
Saturated Fat	3g	Saturated Fat	9g
Sodium	678mg	Sodium	163mg
Cholesterol	89mg	Cholesterol	82mg
Calories	260	Calories	488

FABULOUS MASHED POTATOES
serves 6–8

3 pounds baking or Yukon Gold (available seasonally) potatoes,
    peeled and cut into 1 inch chunks
6–8 garlic cloves, peeled
1/2 cup coarsely chopped celery
1/2 cup nonfat sour cream
1 (3 ounce) package nonfat cream cheese
1/2 cup skim milk, heated
salt and freshly ground black pepper

Place the potatoes, garlic and the celery in a large pan of enough
cold, lightly salted water to cover the potatoes. Bring to a boil, reduce the heat, cover and simmer about 30 minutes. Drain and return to the pan.

    With a handheld electric mixer or whip, beat the potatoes over
low heat until light and fluffy. Add the nonfat sour cream, nonfat
cream cheese and skim milk and continue to whip to incorporate
all of the milk. (Beating the potatoes over a low heat helps to "dry
out" the potatoes of any excess water and allows them to be
"fluffed" to their fullest). Season to taste with salt and pepper.
Serve at once.

Nutrition Analysis
1 Cup

Fabulous Mashed Potatoes	Traditional Mashed Potatoes
Fat 0g	Fat 7g
Saturated Fat 0g	Saturated Fat 1g
Sodium 74mg	Sodium 364mg
Cholesterol 0mg	Cholesterol 0mg
Calories 180	Calories 229

BAKED MACARONI AND CHEESE

serves 8

1 tablespoon reduced fat margarine
1 tablespoon flour
salt and freshly ground black pepper to taste
2 cups skim milk
1 1/2 cups shredded reduced fat cheddar cheese, divided
4 cups cooked elbow macaroni
1/4 cup reduced fat seasoned breadcrumbs

Preheat the oven to 350 degrees. In a medium saucepan melt the margarine, add the flour and the salt and pepper to taste. Cook over low heat, stirring all the time until mixture is smooth and bubbly. Add the skim milk, bring to a boil and cook for one minute. Remove from the heat and add 1 cup of the cheese, stirring until it is melted and smooth. In a large bowl toss the cooked macaroni with the cheese sauce. Set aside.

Lightly coat an 8 x 12 inch baking dish with vegetable spray. Transfer the macaroni to the prepared dish. Top with the remaining shredded cheese and breadcrumbs. Bake in the preheated 350 degree oven until hot and bubbly and a golden crust has formed on the top, about 30 minutes.

Note: For a main meal casserole, stir in 2 cups cooked shredded chicken.

Nutrition Analysis
1 Cup

Baked Macaroni and Cheese	Traditional Macaroni and Cheese
Fat 1g	Fat 17g
Saturated Fat 0g	Saturated Fat 8g
Sodium 222mg	Sodium 687mg
Cholesterol 1mg	Cholesterol 34mg
Calories 176	Calories 328

HOT AND SPICY TURKEY CHILI
serves 8

1 pound lean ground turkey
1 onion, chopped
4 garlic cloves, chopped
2 tablespoons chili powder
1 tablespoon ground cumin
$1/2$ tsp cayenne pepper (optional)
1 (28 ounce) can chopped tomatoes with their juice
1 (15 $1/2$ ounce) can white beans, rinsed and drained
1 (15 $1/2$) can black beans, rinsed and drained
1 (15 $1/2$ ounce) can creamed corn
2 tablespoons Nonfat sour cream
1 tablespoon shredded reduced fat cheddar cheese
salt and freshly ground black pepper to taste

In a large skillet cook the ground turkey, onion and garlic until the turkey is no longer pink and has broken up into small pieces, about 8 minutes. Drain off the excess fat and discard. Stir in the chili powder, cumin and optional cayenne pepper. Add the chopped tomatoes and their juices, the white beans, black beans and creamed corn. Simmer, uncovered for 45–50 minutes or until thickened. Taste and adjust the seasonings with salt and pepper.

Serve immediately with small dollops of nonfat sour cream and a sprinkling of the shredded reduced fat cheese on top.

Note: This turkey chili freezes beautifully for 3 months. Extra lean (93 % lean) ground beef can be substituted for the ground turkey.

Nutrition Analysis
$1^1/2$ Cups

Hot and Spicy Turkey Chili	Traditional Chili
Fat 6g	Fat 24g
Saturated Fat 2g	Saturated Fat 12g
Sodium 720mg	Sodium 478mg
Cholesterol 56mg	Cholesterol 100mg
Calories 218	Calories 428

BRAISED VEGETABLE BEEF STEW
serves 12

2 teaspoons olive oil
1 pound bottom round steak, trimmed of all visible fat,
    cut into 1" cubes
3 cups low sodium beef broth
1/4 cup balsamic vinegar
1/4 cup Dijon mustard
1 (15 1/2 ounce) can chopped tomatoes with their juice
1 (10 3/4 ounce) can low fat cream of celery soup
2 onions, peeled and quartered
4 garlic cloves, peeled and thinly sliced
3 carrots, peeled and cut into 1" pieces
3 ribs of celery, cut on the diagonal into 1" pieces
8 small new potatoes, scrubbed and cut in half
2 tablespoons freshly chopped rosemary or 1 tablespoon dried
    Italian seasoning
salt and freshly ground black pepper

In a Dutch oven or deep skillet heat the olive oil until sizzling. Add
the steak and brown on all sides. Transfer the meat to a plate. With
a paper towel, wipe the Dutch oven or skillet clean.

Stir in the broth, balsamic vinegar, mustard, chopped tomatoes,
celery soup, onions, garlic, carrots, celery, new potatoes, rosemary
or dried Italian seasoning and salt and pepper to taste. Bring to a
boil, add the meat to the Dutch oven/skillet, reduce the heat to
medium low, cover with a tight fitting lid and simmer, stirring every
20 minutes to prevent sticking for 1 to 1 1/2 hours or until stew is
thickened. Transfer to a serving platter and serve at once.

Nutrition Analysis
1 Cup

Braised Vegetable Beef Stew	Traditional Beef Stew
Fat 7g	Fat 12g
Saturated Fat 2g	Saturated Fat 5g
Sodium 222mg	Sodium 335mg
Cholesterol 24mg	Cholesterol 82mg
Calories 147	Calories 253

GUILTLESS CAESAR SALAD
serves 8

3 garlic cloves, peeled
3 anchovy fillets (optional), drained and patted dry
2 tablespoons Dijon mustard
1/2 cup frozen egg substitute, defrosted
1/3 cup red wine vinegar
1 tablespoon Worcestershire sauce
2 cups nonfat sour cream alternative
2 heads Romaine lettuce, washed and separated into leaves or
    torn into bite sized pieces
1 cup fat free shredded Parmesan cheese
2 cups toasted fat free seasoned croutons or fat free store bought
    salt and freshly ground black pepper

In a food processor combine the garlic cloves, optional anchovies and capers until well blended, like a paste. Add the mustard and egg substitute, vinegar and Worcestershire sauce. Blend until smooth. Slowly beat or whisk in the sour cream alternative until thick and creamy.

In a large serving bowl, toss the Romaine with the dressing, shredded Parmesan cheese, croutons, and salt and pepper to taste. Serve at once.

Nutrition Analysis
2 Cups

Guiltless Caesar Salad	Traditional Caesar Salad
Fat 1g	Fat . . . . 54g(!)
Saturated Fat 0g	Saturated Fat 10g
Sodium 482mg	Sodium 987mg
Cholesterol 9mg	Cholesterol 155mg
Calories 131	Calories 620

HEART HEALTHY FETTUCCINE ALFREDO
makes 8 one-cup servings

2 tablespoons reduced fat margarine
4 garlic cloves, chopped
2 tablespoons all purpose flour
3 cups skim milk
1 (8 ounce) package nonfat cream cheese, cubed and softened
2 cups freshly grated Parmesan cheese
8 cups hot cooked fettuccine, cooked without any additional fat or
    salt
2 tablespoons freshly chopped parsley (optional)
Freshly cracked black pepper to taste

In a medium saucepan over low heat, melt the margarine, add the chopped garlic and cook, stirring constantly for about 2 minutes. Stir in the flour and cook for 1 minute more. Gradually add the skim milk whisking until thoroughly blended. Raise the heat to medium and cook for about 8 minutes or until the mixture is thick and bubbly.

Stir in the nonfat cream cheese and cook for 2 minutes. Add 1 1/2 cups of the Parmesan cheese, stirring constantly until the cheese melts. Pour the sauce over the hot cooked pasta and toss to coat evenly. Place the fettuccine on a large serving platter and top with the remaining Parmesan cheese, chopped parsley and the cracked pepper. Serve at once.

Nutrition Analysis
1 Cup

Heart Healthy Fettuccine Alfredo	Traditional Fettuccine Alfredo
Fat 11g	Fat 34g
Saturated Fat 6g	Saturated Fat 14g
Sodium 602mg	Sodium 413mg
Cholesterol 80mg	Cholesterol 119mg
Calories 402	Calories 544

VEGETABLE AND CHEESE LASAGNA
serves 8

2 onions, chopped
4 garlic cloves, chopped
2 yellow squash, halved lengthwise and thinly sliced
2 zucchini, halved lengthwise and thinly sliced
1/4 cup balsamic vinegar
1 (28 ounce) can chopped plum tomatoes, with their juice
1 (6 ounce) can tomato paste
1 cup water
1/4 cup freshly chopped basil
1 tablespoon dried Italian seasoning
2 teaspoons fennel seed

salt and freshly ground black pepper
1 tablespoon sugar
1 (24 ounce container) fat free cottage cheese, drained
1/2 cup egg substitute
1/2 cup freshly grated Parmesan cheese
1 cup reduced fat grated mozzarella cheese
1/2 cup breadcrumbs
12 lasagna noodles, cooked according to package directions
1/4 cup freshly grated Parmesan cheese

In a large saucepan combine the onions, garlic, yellow squash, zucchini, balsamic vinegar, plum tomatoes, tomato paste, water, basil, dried Italian seasoning, fennel seed, and the sugar. Salt and pepper to taste. Bring to a boil, reduce the heat to a simmer and cook for 30–40 minutes or until sauce is thickened. Be sure to stir every now and then to prevent the sauce from sticking.

Meanwhile, in a large bowl, combine the cottage cheese, egg substitute, Parmesan cheese, mozzarella cheese and the bread crumbs. Mix well and set aside.

Lightly coat a 13x9x2 inch baking dish with vegetable spray. Place a single layer of the pasta on the bottom of the dish (about 4 strips). Cover with 1/3 of the tomato sauce and then half of the cottage cheese mixture. Top the cottage cheese mixture with another layer of pasta, add 1/3 more of the sauce and the rest of the cheese mixture. To finish, place a final layer of pasta on top, cover with the remaining tomato sauce and top this with the Parmesan cheese.

Place in a preheated 400 degree oven and cook until heated through and bubbly, about 45 minutes. Let the lasagna sit for 10 minutes before slicing and serving. This dish freezes well.

Note: One large eggplant, cut into cubes can be substituted for the yellow squash and zucchini. Or substitute 1 pound browned and drained extra lean (93% lean) ground beef or turkey if a meat lasagna is desired. This is also a wonderful sauce ladled over hot cooked spaghetti or fettuccine.

Nutrition Analysis
1 3/4 Cups

Vegetable & Cheese Lasagna		Traditional Lasagna	
Fat	4g	Fat	29g
Saturated Fat	2g	Saturated Fat	14g
Sodium	825mg	Sodium	1228mg
Cholesterol	8mg	Cholesterol	75mg
Calories	291	Calories	544

ITALIAN MACARONI AND TURKEY CASSEROLE
serves 6–8

1 pound lean ground turkey
1 onion, chopped
2 garlic cloves, chopped
1 (15¹/2 ounce) can no salt added, diced stewed tomatoes, undrained
1 (10³/4 ounce) can tomato soup
1 tablespoon dried Italian seasoning
¹/4 cup freshly chopped parsley (optional)
4 cups cooked elbow macaroni
1 (15¹/2 ounce) can kidney beans, rinsed and drained
salt and freshly ground black pepper to taste

Preheat the oven to 375 degrees. In a large skillet over medium high heat, cook the ground turkey with the onion and the garlic until the meat is browned and the vegetables are soft, about 5–7 minutes.

Transfer the contents of the skillet to a large bowl and stir in the tomatoes, tomato soup, Italian seasoning, optional parsley, cooked macaroni and kidney beans. Season to taste with salt and pepper.

Place into a large baking pan that has been lightly coated with vegetable spray. Cover tightly with aluminum foil and place in the preheated oven. Bake for 30 minutes or until heated through. Serve at once.

Nutrition Analysis
1¹/2 Cups

Italian Macaroni and Turkey Casserole	Popular boxed mix with regular hamburger
Fat 6g	Fat 17g
Saturated Fat 1g	Saturated Fat 6g
Sodium 500mg	Sodium 1395mg
Cholesterol 62mg	Cholesterol 75mg
Calories 314	Calories 435

BAKED CHICKEN BREASTS WITH CREAMY MUSTARD SAUCE
serves 5

2 tablespoons mustard seed
1/4 cup apple cider vinegar
1/4 cup Dijon mustard
2 tablespoons lemon juice
1/2 cup fat free mayonnaise (can be reduced fat)
3 green onions, finely chopped
2 tablespoon freshly chopped basil or 1 tablespoon Italian Seasoning
5 boneless, skinless chicken breasts
1/2 cup reduced fat seasoned breadcrumbs
1/4 cup grated Parmesan cheese
salt and freshly ground black pepper to taste

Preheat the oven to 400 degrees. Lightly coat a large baking dish with nonstick vegetable spray. Set aside.

In a medium bowl combine the mustard seeds and the apple cider vinegar. Soak for 30 minutes. Add the Dijon mustard, lemon juice, fat free mayonnaise, green onions, basil or dried Italian seasoning, and salt and pepper to taste. Spoon and evenly spread the mustard mixture over the chicken. Sprinkle with the breadcrumbs and Parmesan cheese.

Bake for 25–30 minutes or until chicken is cooked all the way through and the mustard glaze has just begun to brown. Serve at once.

Variation for fish: Substitute 4 (4–6 ounce) tuna or salmon steaks for the chicken. Omit the basil and Parmesan cheese. Add 3 tablespoons of freshly chopped dill and 1 tablespoon capers to the mustard glaze. Bake at 400 degrees for 15–20 minutes or until the fish flakes easily with a fork.

Nutrition Analysis
1 Chicken Breast

Baked Chicken Breast with Creamy Mustard Sauce	Traditional Fried Chicken Breast
Fat 7g	Fat 32g
Saturated Fat 2g	Saturated Fat 9g
Sodium 604mg	Sodium 682mg
Cholesterol 106mg	Cholesterol 210mg
Calories 312	Calories 644

Southwestern Seasoned Rice with Ground Beef

serves 6–8

1 pound extra lean (93% lean) ground beef (or lean ground turkey)
1 onion, chopped
2 garlic cloves, chopped
2 cups long grain rice
1 (15 1/2 ounce) can chopped tomatoes with their juice
1 tablespoon chili powder
1 teaspoon ground cumin
3 cups low sodium beef or chicken broth
1/4 cup freshly chopped cilantro (optional)
1 (15 1/2 ounce) can black beans, rinsed and drained
salt and freshly ground black pepper to taste

Preheat the oven to 375 degrees. In a large skillet over medium high heat, cook the ground beef (or turkey) with the onion and the garlic until the meat is browned and the vegetables are soft, about 5–7 minutes. Drain any excess fat and discard. Add the rice, tomatoes, chili powder and cumin and cook, stirring constantly about 3 minutes longer. Stir in the beef broth (or chicken broth), optional cilantro and the black beans. Season to taste with salt and pepper.

Transfer the contents of the skillet to a large baking pan that has been coated with vegetable spray.

Cover tightly with aluminum foil and place in the preheated oven. Bake for 40 minutes or until all the liquid has been absorbed. Serve at once.

Note: For an entirely vegetarian entree, omit the ground beef and substitute vegetable broth for the beef or chicken broth.

Nutrition Analysis
1 1/2 Cups

Southwestern Seasoned Rice with Ground Beef	Traditional Rice and Ground Beef
Fat 10g	Fat 17g
Saturated Fat 4g	Saturated Fat 3g
Sodium 423mg	Sodium 698mg
Cholesterol 40mg	Cholesterol 73mg
Calories 259	Calories 414

BETTER BEEF STROGANOFF
serves 8

1 pound very lean boneless sirloin steak, thinly sliced
salt and freshly ground black pepper to taste
1 onion, chopped
1 green or red pepper, seeded and thinly sliced
2 carrots, peeled and shredded
4 garlic cloves, chopped
2 teaspoons canola oil
2 teaspoons flour
1 1/2 cups low sodium chicken or beef broth
1 tablespoon Worcestershire sauce
2 teaspoons dry mustard
1 tablespoon dried thyme
1 (8 ounce) containers nonfat sour cream
1 (8 ounce) package) nonfat cream cheese
1 tablespoon cornstarch
5 cups cooked medium nonfat egg noodles, cooked without added salt or fat
4 green onions, chopped

Lightly season the sliced steak with salt and pepper. Lightly spray a large Dutch oven with the vegetable spray. Add the steak, onion, green or red pepper, carrots and garlic. Cook over medium heat until the steak is browned and the vegetables are tender, about 10 minutes.

Remove the contents of the pan to a large bowl and set aside. In the same Dutch oven, over medium heat, heat the canola oil and add the flour, stirring constantly until you have a light brown roux, about 1–2 minutes. Add the broth and cook until the mixture reduces by half, about 10 minutes.

In a food processor or blender combine the Worcestershire sauce, dry mustard, thyme, nonfat sour cream, nonfat cream cheese and cornstarch until smooth. Add this to the reduced broth mixture and stir constantly, just until the mixture comes to a boil. Stir in the sautéed meat and vegetables. Cook until just heated through, 2–3 minutes. Spread the cooked egg noodles on a large serving platter. Spoon the meat sauce over the egg noodles and top with the chopped green onions.

Nutrition Analysis
1 1/2 Cups

Better Beef Stroganoff	Traditional Beef Stroganoff
Fat 7g	Fat 37g
Saturated Fat 2g	Saturated Fat 13g
Sodium 554mg	Sodium 1519mg
Cholesterol 84mg	Cholesterol 109mg
Calories 350	Calories 626

TURKEY FAJITAS
serves 4–6

8 (8 inch) flour tortillas
1 tablespoon chili powder
2 teaspoons ground cumin
1/4 teaspoon cayenne pepper
    (optional)
1 pound turkey breast cutlets,
    pounded thin between two
    pieces of plastic wrap
1 teaspoon canola or vegetable oil
1 red pepper, seeded and thinly
    sliced
1 green pepper, seeded and
    thinly sliced

1 red onion, peeled and thinly
    sliced
3 garlic cloves, peeled and thinly
    sliced
juice of 1 lime
salt and freshly ground black
    pepper to taste
2 tablespoons nonfat sour cream
1 tablespoon shredded reduced fat
    cheddar cheese

Garnishes: shredded lettuce,
    chopped tomatoes

Preheat the oven to 425 degrees. Wrap all eight of the tortillas together in foil and set aside. On a piece of waxed paper mix together the chili powder, cumin and optional cayenne. With your fingers, rub this mixture into the turkey cutlets. Place on a baking sheet that has been lightly coated with vegetable spray. Place in the oven and cook about 6–8 minutes per side. Remove and set aside. Reduce the oven temperature to 250 degrees and place the wrapped tortillas in the oven to heat.

In a large non-stick skillet, heat the oil until hot. Add the red pepper, green pepper, red onion and garlic. Cook until the peppers are softened and the onion begins to wilt. Stir in the lime juice and salt and pepper to taste. Slice the roasted turkey into thin strips. Mix the turkey into the vegetables and toss over medium heat for one minute. Transfer the mixture to a large serving platter. Top each tortilla with the assorted garnishes, the turkey/vegetable mixture and serve with the Pineapple Salsa, if desired.

Nutrition Analysis
1 Fajita

Turkey Fajitas		Traditional Fajitas	
Fat	5g	Fat	16g
Saturated Fat	1g	Saturated Fat	6g
Sodium	497mg	Sodium	501mg
Cholesterol	41mg	Cholesterol	52mg
Calories	219	Calories	322

PINEAPPLE SALSA
makes about 2 cups

1 (16 ounce can) chopped pineapple in its own juice, drained
2 tablespoons freshly chopped cilantro
1 jalapeno pepper, seeded and finely chopped
Juice of 1 lime
1 teaspoon ground cumin
1 teaspoon chili powder

In a large bowl mix together the chopped pineapple, cilantro, jalapeno pepper, lime juice, cumin and chili powder. Cover and chill for one hour.

Nutrition Analysis
1/2 Cup

Pineapple Salsa	Traditional Salsa
Fat 0g	Fat 0g
Saturated Fat 0g	Saturated Fat 0g
Sodium 39mg	Sodium 456mg
Cholesterol 0mg	Cholesterol 0mg
Calories 35	Calories 13

COMPANY SALMON CAKES
makes approximately eighteen 3 ounce cakes

Vegetable cooking spray
1 teaspoon vegetable oil
2 green onions, finely chopped
2 garlic cloves, chopped
1 small red pepper, seeded and
    finely chopped
1/4 cup apple juice
1 1/2 cups reduced fat seasoned
    breadcrumbs, divided
3 egg whites
2 tablespoons freshly chopped
    parsley

2 teaspoons Old Bay seasoning or
    other seafood seasoning
freshly ground black pepper to taste
1/3 cup nonfat mayonnaise
juice and grated zest of 1 lemon, no
    white attached
1 tablespoon Worcestershire sauce
2 (15 1/2 ounce) cans of salmon,
    drained. Mix with fork for consis-
    tency. Simply mash bones with a
    fork—don't discard—they are a
    great source of calcium.

Preheat the oven to 400 degrees. Lightly coat a baking sheet with vegetable spray and set aside.

Coat a large nonstick skillet with the cooking spray, add the oil and heat over medium high heat until hot. Add the green onions, garlic, and red pepper, reduce the heat to medium and cook until crisp tender, about 3–4 minutes. Add the apple juice and continue cooking until the liquid has evaporated.

Transfer the vegetable mixture to a large bowl and stir in 3/4 cup of the bread crumbs with the egg whites. Stir to mix well. Add the parsley, seafood seasoning, pepper to taste, nonfat mayonnaise, lemon juice and zest and the Worcestershire sauce. Stir in the salmon and combine well.

Shape the salmon mixture into 18 (1" diameter) patties, using about 2 table-spoons mixture per patty. Dredge the patties in the reserved breadcrumbs, cover and chill for 30 minutes.

Place the patties in the preheated 400 degree oven and bake for 10 minutes, turn the crab cakes over and bake for 10 minutes more, or until heated through and nicely browned. Serve warm or at room temperature with Fat Free Tartar Sauce, if desired.

Nutrition Analysis
1 Salmon Cake

Company Salmon Cakes		Traditional Salmon Cakes	
Fat	4g	Fat	7g
Saturated Fat	0g	Saturated Fat	1g
Sodium	578mg	Sodium	270mg
Cholesterol	12mg	Cholesterol	40mg
Calories	120	Calories	126

Note: Although there's not much difference between the Company and the Traditional recipes, it's been included so that you'll have something a little different and nice to serve your guests. I personally eat a lot of canned salmon—you and your family would probably do well to eat more yourself. It's convenient, inexpensive, and tastes great too. For an even simpler recipe, try the *Salmon Burgers* on the following page.

SALMON BURGERS
Makes 4 salmon burgers

1 15 ½ oz. can salmon
2 egg whites
½ cup breadcrumbs
½ cup chopped onion
½ cup chopped green pepper
1 T lemon juice
1 T grated lemon peel
½ t dill
⅛ t pepper

Drain the salmon and flake. Combine the ingredients, mix well and form into four patties. Pan-fry in about 2 tablespoons of light olive oil until lightly browned on both sides.

Serve on toasted hamburger buns. Top with ketchup, Dijon mustard, or fat free tartar sauce.

Nutrition Analysis
1 Salmon Burger with Bun

Salmon Burger with Bun	Traditional Hamburger with Bun
Fat 9g	Fat 21g
Saturated Fat 2g	Saturated Fat 8g
Sodium 927mg	Sodium 660mg
Cholesterol 57mg	Cholesterol 86mg
Calories 326	Calories 410

CHOCOLATE MOIST 'N CHEWY BROWNIES
makes 24 brownies

2 cups all purpose flour
2 cups confectioners sugar
2/3 cup cocoa powder
2 teaspoons baking powder
1/2 teaspoon cinnamon
1/4 cup whipped reduced fat margarine, melted
1 cup packed brown sugar
1/4 cup light corn syrup
2 tablespoons skim milk
1 tablespoon vanilla
1/2 cup egg substitute
Confectioners sugar for dusting

Preheat the oven to 350 degrees. Lightly coat an 8 x12" baking pan with vegetable spray. Set aside.

In a large bowl sift together the flour, confectioners sugar, cocoa, baking powder, and cinnamon. Set aside. In a medium bowl combine the melted margarine, brown sugar, corn syrup, skim milk, vanilla and egg substitute. Stir the wet ingredients into the dry ingredients and mix until well combined.

Transfer the batter to the prepared pan. Bake in the preheated oven 26–28 minutes, or until the center of the brownies are almost firm when touched and beginning to pull away from the sides of the pan. Remove to a wire rack and cool completely (at least 2 hours) before cutting into squares. Dust with the confectioners sugar and place on a serving platter or cake stand. These freeze very well, tightly wrapped for 3 months.

Nutrition Analysis
1 Brownie

Chocolate Moist 'n' Chewy Brownies	Traditional Brownies
Fat 2g	Fat 7g
Saturated Fat 0g	Saturated Fat 2g
Sodium 40mg	Sodium 132mg
Cholesterol 0mg	Cholesterol 8mg
Calories 135	Calories 172

CHOCOLATE ANGEL FOOD CAKE
makes one (10 inch) tube cake, 10 servings

1¼ cups cake flour or Southern soft wheat flour (such as White Lily)
1¼ cups sugar, divided
⅓ cup Dutch processed cocoa powder
½ teaspoon cinnamon
14 large egg whites
1½ teaspoons cream of tartar
¼ teaspoons salt
1 tablespoon vanilla extract
½ cup mini semisweet chocolate chips
Confectioners sugar
Freshly sliced strawberries (optional)

Preheat the oven to 375 degrees. Sift the flour, 1/4 cup of the sugar, cocoa powder and the cinnamon together on a piece of waxed paper. Repeat sifting process two more times. Set aside.

In a large mixing bowl beat together the egg whites, cream of tartar and salt until soft peaks form. Gradually beat in the remaining 1 cup of sugar (about 1/4 cup at a time) until very stiff peaks form. Beat in the vanilla extract.

Sift about 1/4 of the flour/cocoa mixture over the top of the whites. Gently fold this into the beaten whites. Repeat this process 3 more times, using the rest of the flour/cocoa. Fold in the mini chocolate chips. Spoon or ladle the chocolate batter into a 10" *ungreased* tube pan with removable bottom. Run a knife or spatula gently through the batter to eliminate any air pockets. Bake in the lower third of the oven until lightly browned, about 35–40 minutes.

Invert the pan to cool completely. When cool, run a thin knife or spatula around the edges of the cake to loosen. Turn the cake onto a serving platter. Sprinkle with confectioners sugar and garnish and serve with fresh strawberry slices if desired.

VARIATION: To make a plain angel food cake, simply omit the cocoa powder, cinnamon and the chocolate chips. Add 1 tablespoon freshly squeezed lemon juice and 1/2 teaspoon almond extract with the vanilla.

Nutrition Analysis
1 Slice

Chocolate Angel Food Cake		Traditional Boxed Chocolate Cake with Frosting	
Fat	4g	Fat	12g
Saturated Fat	2g	Saturated Fat	6g
Sodium	130mg	Sodium	262mg
Cholesterol	0mg	Cholesterol	54mg
Calories	234	Calories	341

CHOCOLATE SWIRL CHEESECAKE
makes 1 (10") cheesecake, 12 servings

1¹/2 cups graham cracker crumbs
¹/4 cup reduced fat margarine, melted
3 tablespoons sugar
1 (16 ounce) carton part skim ricotta cheese, drained
2 (8 ounce) packages nonfat cream cheese, softened
1 (8 ounce) carton nonfat sour cream

1 cup sugar
3 tablespoons all purpose flour
2 teaspoons vanilla extract
³/4 cup egg substitute
2 tablespoons cocoa powder
1 tablespoon reduced fat margarine, melted
Sliced strawberries for garnish

Preheat the oven to 350 degrees. In a small bowl combine the graham cracker crumbs, melted margarine and the sugar. Press the mixture into the bottom of a 10" springform pan. Bake at 350 degrees for 10–12 minutes. Remove from the oven and cool completely.

Meanwhile, in a food processor or mixer combine the ricotta cheese, nonfat cream cheese, nonfat sour cream, sugar and flour. Mix until smooth. Add the vanilla and egg substitute. Mix until well combined. Reserve 1 cup of this mixture. Pour the remaining mixture into the prepared crust.

In a small bowl combine the cocoa and the melted margarine. Stir until smooth. Add the reserved cheesecake mixture and stir just to blend. Drizzle this mixture over the cheesecake mixture in the pan. With a knife, swirl the chocolate into the vanilla mixture creating a marbled effect.

Place the pan in the preheated oven, reduce the heat to 325 degrees and bake for 15 minutes. Reduce the oven temperature to 250 degrees and bake for 60–70 minutes longer. Turn off the oven and let the cheesecake cool in the oven for 3 hours longer. Remove from the oven and let cool on a wire rack.

Cover and chill in the refrigerator 8 hours or overnight. When ready to serve, loosen the edge of the pan with a knife or a spatula and unmold the cheesecake. Place on a serving platter and garnish with sliced strawberries if desired.

Note: For a plain cheesecake simply omit the cocoa powder and reduced fat margarine from the swirling process. Increase the vanilla extract by 1 tablespoon.

Nutrition Analysis
1 Slice

Chocolate Swirl Cheesecake	Traditional Cheesecake
Fat 7g	Fat 32g
Saturated Fat 3g	Saturated Fat 15g
Sodium 345mg	Sodium 403mg
Cholesterol 12mg	Cholesterol 118mg
Calories 246	Calories 501

PERFECT PUMPKIN PIE
serves 8

$3/4$ cup packed brown sugar
$1/4$ cup all purpose flour
2 teaspoons cinnamon
1 teaspoon ground ginger
$1/4$ teaspoon ground cloves
$1/8$ teaspoon freshly grated nutmeg
$1/2$ teaspoon salt
$1/2$ cup egg substitute
1 teaspoon vanilla extract
1 (15 ounce) can solid pack pumpkin (*not pumpkin pie filling*)
1 (12 ounce) can evaporated skim milk (*not sweetened condensed milk*)
1 unbaked 9" deep dish pie shell (preferably one made with vegetable shortening)

Preheat the oven to 425 degrees. In a large bowl mix together the brown sugar, flour, cinnamon, ginger, cloves, nutmeg, salt, egg substitute, vanilla and pumpkin. Slowly whisk in the evaporated skim milk until smooth.

Pour into the prepared pie shell and bake in the preheated oven for 15 minutes. Reduce the temperature to 350 degrees and continue baking for an additional 40–50 minutes or until a knife inserted into the center of the pie comes out clean. Cool on a wire rack for at least 2 hours.

Nutrition Analysis
1 slice

Perfect Pumpkin Pie		Traditional Pumpkin Pie	
Fat	.6g	Fat	.14g
Saturated Fat	.1g	Saturated Fat	.5g
Sodium	.317mg	Sodium	.349mg
Cholesterol	.1mg	Cholesterol	.65mg
Calories	.246	Calories	.316

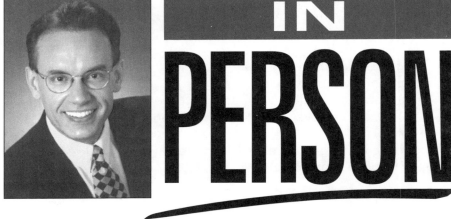

DAVID MEINZ IN PERSON

Invite David Meinz to bring one of his programs to your church, business or association. Contact:

David Meinz, MS, RD, FADA, CSP
1-407-854-8108
PO Box 772525, Orlando, FL 32877

Be sure to visit our web site at
www.DavidMeinz.com